Thyroid Disorders and
Related Health Conditions

Eight Intriguing Sections on
the Metabolic Butterfly

By: James M. Lowrance   Revised Version © 2020

I0416474

This Eight Section book (Approx. 70,375 words in length) is comprehensive about thyroid disorders and health conditions that are strongly related to them. Symptoms are discussed, as well as diagnostic and treatment methods -- both medical and natural. The reader will find out about the most effective treatments available for thyroid diseases, including facts about how thyroid hormone therapy can be tweaked and optimized for best possible results. Other health conditions that are strongly associated with thyroid problems, are also discussed, including joint/muscle pain, chronic fatigue, emotional disorders and fatigued adrenal glands. This is a very large resource containing 104 Chapters. Page numbers are shown for each section, so that a reader can go to specific subjects when needed.

MAIN TABLE OF SECTIONS:

⍰

SECTION ONE

Hypothyroid and Hyperthyroid Disorders

TABLE OF CONTENTS:

11. My Review for - Hypothyroidism Type 2: The Epidemic

1. A Simple Look at Hypothyroidism Causes

Having hypothyroidism means your thyroid gland is underactive. When this occurs, your bodily metabolism is slowed down. What causes this condition to develop both commonly and uncommonly?

Hypothyroidism can be caused by several different things but in the more industrialized countries of the world, the cause is "thyroid autoimmunity", also called "autoimmune thyroiditis" and "Hashimoto's disease".

How Thyroid Autoimmunity Occurs

Thyroid autoimmunity is a disease-process in which the thyroid gland becomes under-active, after being relentlessly attacked by auto-antibodies sent from the immune system that mistakenly identify it as an intruder to the body, as it would allergens, bacteria and viruses. Once enough thyroid cells are damaged by these antibodies over time, hypothyroidism sets in as a result of less healthy tissue being present within the thyroid gland. It can no longer continue manufacturing thyroid hormones, at the rate the body needs them, and symptoms of a low metabolism will begin to occur. One possibility that has been considered for the high percent of hypothyroid cases in this category, is the increase in environmental toxins existing in the world today, which have a negative impact upon the immune system, causing it to malfunction in its duty to protect the body from illness-causing invaders.

Most-Common and Least-Common Causes of Underactive Thyroids

In the less industrialized countries of the world (our largest populations), where iodine rich foods are lacking or they do not have access to iodized table salt, as we do who live in the wealthier nations, "Iodine Deficiency Hypothyroidism" can be the cause of underactive thyroid glands. It is in fact, the number one cause of underactive thyroid glands, worldwide. The least common cause of hypothyroid conditions is a failure within the brain glands that regulate thyroid function (master endocrine gland failure) which is called "Central Hypothyroidism". The two glands that are first affected in cases of Central Hypothyroidism, are the "hypothalamus and/or the pituitary". One or both of these glands, will develop malignant or benign tumors within them, resulting in this relatively rare condition. This cause of hypothyroid conditions represents less than one percent of all cases, worldwide.

Thyroid Dysfunction in Birthing

Women can develop a temporary form of thyroiditis after they become pregnant, that will afterward leave them hypothyroid, called "Postpartum Hypothyroidism". If hypothyroidism begins during pregnancy, it may be referred to as "gestational hypothyroidism". In some cases, the resulting underactive thyroid is temporary and other times it is permanent, needing lifelong treatment. This is because pregnancy can bring permanent thyroid autoimmunity to the surface in some women. Some people are born with insufficient thyroid glands (small or partially missing) and as they enter their preteens or teen years, their thyroid hormone levels become inadequate. This is referred to as "Juvenile Hypothyroidism" but in some cases it is diagnosed at birth and treated, with no negative consequences as the child develops, which is then referred to as "Congenital Hypothyroidism". If it is the congenital type, this means it does not continue to run a course, once treated shortly after birth.

Thyroid Failure from Injury and Chemicals

People who experience severe throat injuries, such as those that can occur with car accidents, can damage their thyroid glands to the extent that they become underactive and lastly, a person can experience hypothyroidism following exposure to chemicals or drugs that adversely affect the thyroid gland, called "Chemical Hypothyroidism". Lots of Russian people experienced Chemical Hypothyroidism following the Chernobyl nuclear power plant accident in 1986, in which nuclear fallout affected their thyroid glands in years following, causing them to become under active. For this reason, it is highly recommended for people who work in radiology imaging labs and for medical and dental patients receiving x-rays, to wear protective clothing or gear, that prevents radioactivity from being absorbed into their bodies, in higher amounts than are absolutely necessary. At the basic level, an under active thyroid simply means one that is not producing enough hormone to properly regulate bodily metabolism. It is a treatable condition, requiring thyroid hormone replacement therapy, to restore bodily metabolism to normal levels.

People who experience severe throat injuries, such as those that can occur with car accidents, can damage their thyroid glands to the extent that they become underactive and lastly, a person can experience hypothyroidism following exposure to chemicals or drugs that adversely affect the thyroid gland, called "Chemical Hypothyroidism". Lots of Russian people experienced Chemical Hypothyroidism following the Chernobyl nuclear power plant accident in 1986, in which nuclear fallout affected their thyroid glands in years following, causing them to become under active. For this reason, it is highly recommended for people who work in radiology imaging labs and for medical and dental patients receiving x-rays, to wear protective clothing or gear, that prevents radioactivity from being absorbed into their bodies, in higher amounts than are absolutely necessary. At the basic level, an under active thyroid simply means one that is not producing enough hormone to properly regulate bodily metabolism. It is a treatable condition, requiring thyroid hormone replacement therapy, to restore bodily metabolism to normal levels.

At the basic level, an under active thyroid simply means one that is not producing enough hormone to properly regulate bodily metabolism. It is a treatable condition, requiring thyroid hormone replacement therapy, to restore bodily metabolism to normal levels.

2. Antibodies a Cause of Hypothyroid Symptoms

Sometime ago, I had an office visit with an Endocrinologist, and I took my LabOne blood test results with me. He found on the results, where my thyroid hormone levels were at optimal range (Free T-3 at top of normal) but even though I had been on hormone replacement medication (Armour), for over two years, my TG and TPO antibodies were still elevated. My Anti-TG ABs (Anti-Thyroglobulin), were "537" (normal range <40), so were about 500 points above normal. My Anti-TPO ABs (anti-Thyroid peroxidase), were "120" (normal range <35), so were about 85 points above normal.

My complaint at that time was continuing mild to moderate joint pain, especially in my upper spine and shoulders and moderate, intermittent fatigue. His response to this was that elevated antibody levels also mean there is resulting "inflammation" and that this could cause these symptoms, apart from my normal thyroid hormone levels. I was amazed that other doctors I had seen and even the drug manufacturer's websites, do not mention the role of thyroid antibodies, in causing ongoing symptoms, despite proper hormone replacement medication treatment.

My Endo prescribed me a short-term round of "corticosteroids" (anti-inflammatory steroid) and told me afterward that I could take occasional over-the-counter anti-inflammatory medications like Ibuprofen to help with symptoms. For a period afterward, my joint pain had gone down to only rare, mild occurrence and I rarely had the need to take an anti-inflammatory. Now, a few years later, the arthritic pain returned, as well as chronic fatigue and my belief is that thyroid antibodies, which increased again and remained at high levels, have played a major role in the return of my symptoms.

I am not sure why more is not being expressed in this area because it makes complete sense that highly activated immune system activity, means a bodily response manifesting in different degrees of symptoms, depending upon how highly elevated antibody levels are. Inflammation from the autoimmune disease process also manifests in symptoms, which means the disease process itself is also what causes illness in treated hypothyroid patients and not the resulting hypothyroidism alone.

When patients complain to their doctors about symptoms, but their hormone levels are replaced to optimal levels, the doctor will likely tell the patient that their symptoms cannot be thyroid disease related because their hormone levels have been corrected. I have heard this scenario related by many, many patients however, when these patients ask for a retest of their thyroid antibody levels, they will come back highly elevated. I have heard some patients report TPO levels in the 1,000s which would seem to be a prime candidate for explaining unrelieved symptoms, but some doctors seem to believe the antibodies levels are insignificant.

It is the opinion of much research that has been conducted, that thyroid antibodies do play a role in symptoms and it is my hope that even more research and surveys will be conducted, addressing the symptomology of thyroid antibodies in treated hypothyroid patients.

3. Are Thyroid Disease Patients Complainers?

You may see the title of this article and wonder what in the world could this one be about?! My intention in this article is to bring attention to the fact that thyroid disease symptoms can be very serious and no matter whom they may affect, they can seriously alter a person's life and have a negative impact upon their emotions and quality of life. This includes even the strongest of people who may experience the onset of a thyroid disease.

Over the years I have read the blogs and books of thyroid patients who report that, friends or loved ones believe they are being complainers. In some cases, this was devastating to the person because on top of severe symptom-struggles and feeling as if they are barely surviving their disease, they have someone make such an inconsiderate and non-compassionate remark. I have also read the testimonies of thyroid patients whose marriages crumbled due to the frustration of a spouse who thought their husband or wife was over-reacting to the symptoms of their disease or simply playing on their sympathy and trying to get attention.

If these people with this view that thyroid patients are over-reacting to their symptoms, could step into that person's shoes for just one day, they would gain a completely different understanding. Using myself for an example, before thyroid disease, I was never one to give in when I was sick or allow symptoms to keep me from doing things, including going to work. I remember times working when I had severe flu symptoms, bronchitis and other times when I worked even when I thought I was suffering pneumonia. I made doctor visits probably less than once every five years and I had to be very sick to see one and it usually required that my wife tweak me before I would make a doctor office visit.

I am a pretty big guy at 6 foot, 225 lbs. and I have always been strong and love outdoors sports, but the onset of thyroid disease hit me very hard and I basically buckled under the symptoms of it for a time. I remember after going through a very stressful period, falling into incredibly harsh symptoms that in my case cycled between hypothyroid and hyperthyroid symptoms at first. I would experience incredibly severe fatigue and exhaustion, and this would then phase into extreme panic attacks with profuse sweating and temporary rapid weight loss.

I lost my ability to concentrate and completely lost my appetite for several weeks. The fear of the unknown of what was happening to me, sunk me into a severe state of anxiety and depression, at which time, I finally went to see a doctor. The doctor incorrectly diagnosed me with emotional problems only (which was certainly a part of it) and I had to demand blood testing before the proper diagnosis was made. Even with treatment, I can occasionally fall into mild to moderate spells of symptoms and less-frequently I can experience severe symptoms.

In my case I have a supportive and compassionate family who, have been supporting me from the beginning. I truly wish all thyroid patients had this same benefit but sadly, some do not. I know other strong people who have been seriously affected by thyroid disease symptoms, including a man I am in communication with by phone who also has hypothyroidism caused by Hashimoto's thyroiditis, as I do. He was previously a race car driver and has told me often of the fact that he seldom experienced fear on the track or otherwise. This changed when he experienced the onset of thyroid disease and he has at times gone through serious struggles with the symptoms it has caused him.

Famous athletes have experienced thyroid disease and have gone through severe struggles as well, until they were properly diagnosed and treated. This includes names like Carl Lewis, 10-time Olympic gold winner in track and field and Gail Devers, an Olympic sprinter who also won a gold medal in her sport.

If you are the spouse, loved one or friend of a thyroid disease patient, I implore you to exercise patience, understanding and compassion toward the thyroid patients in your life. This can be greatly instrumental in helping them to benefit more from treatments and in coping with a disease that has greatly affected their lives.

4. Basics about Central Hypothyroidism

The endocrine system (includes the thyroid), is controlled by glands located at the center of the brain. Failures in this system can occur, including hypothyroidism.

For most patients who are diagnosed with hypothyroidism, the cause is a misdirected immune system response called "thyroid autoimmunity", meaning the immune system has turned against the thyroid gland and is sending auto-antibodies (cells that normally destroy germs and allergens), to attack it. The name for the resulting damage and inflammation in the thyroid gland is "Hashimoto's thyroiditis" and a common medical term for the condition is "Chronic Lymphocytic thyroiditis". There is however a non-immune related type of hypothyroidism that is less common, called "Central Hypothyroidism".

With Central Hypothyroidism, the low functioning thyroid gland is a result of inadequate communication between glands within the endocrine system, that normally work together in regulating thyroid function. The hypothalamus and pituitary glands are located within the brain-center and they send signals to other endocrine glands, via hormones that communicate and stimulate other glands, including those sent to the adrenals and to the thyroid.

The hypothalamus is the first gland in the chain of command, which sends a hormone to the pituitary gland, signaling it to release a hormone of its own that is then sent to the thyroid gland, to regulate thyroid hormone production. TRH: "Thyrotropin Releasing Hormone" is the one sent from the hypothalamus to the pituitary gland, which stimulates it to release a thyroid regulating hormone called TSH "Thyroid Stimulating Hormone". The thyroid gland will then respond by producing either thyroid hormones (T4 and T3), according to how much TSH is sent to it. Some medical sources call this the "hypothalamus-pituitary-thyroid axis".

When something goes wrong within this system of glands whose end-purpose is regulating thyroid function, it can cause the thyroid to release inadequate amounts of hormone, resulting in hypothyroidism. If there is disease present in one of the two major brain glands (hypothalamus or pituitary), such as a tumor-adenoma that develops within one of them or damage of some type occurs in one or both of them (such as from traumatic injury), they may fail to regulate the endocrine glands they are in charge of.

A treating physician that diagnosis hypothyroidism in a patient, can determine if the cause is dysfunction in one of these glands, by blood testing the patient's levels of TRH and/or TSH, and/or by ordering brain imaging tests such as an MRI, that checks for the presence of tumors. None of these tests are necessary, if the cause of hypothyroidism is already obvious, such as when a patient tests positive for "thyroid antibodies"(thyroid autoimmunity), which would be a problem originating from within the thyroid gland itself -- also referred to as "primary hypothyroidism".

When a type of hypothyroidism, is not a problem within the thyroid gland itself, it is referred to as a "secondary cause", such as with Central Hypothyroidism. Most patients who are diagnosed with Central Hypothyroidism are first suspected of having it, when their thyroid hormones (T4 and/or T3) are found to be at low, hypothyroid levels but the TSH level is in normal range or actually flagged low at the same. A Low TSH usually indicates hyperthyroidism (overactive) and not hypothyroidism and therefore Central Hypothyroidism is investigated as a possible cause in these cases.

5. Best Results from Thyroid Hormone Therapy

There are simple steps that can be taken, that will help thyroid hormone replacement therapy to work better for patients being treated for hypothyroidism. Optimizing dose-taking practices is the key.

People taking thyroid hormone replacement medication for hypothyroidism need to follow a set routine for taking their medication. Hormone therapy can have a delicate balance; even small variations in the levels created in the body from taking a hormone medication can greatly affect how well a patient feels. The 5 steps below help to insure the best results from thyroid hormone replacement therapy.

1. Take your thyroid hormone medication on an empty stomach, with plenty of water:

Many patients find it easier to take their thyroid medication on an empty stomach by doing so first thing in the morning before having breakfast. Once the medication has been taken, it is recommended that a patient wait at least 30 minutes before eating, to allow the medication time to be absorbed in the digestive tract (waiting an hour is even better). Taking the medication with a full glass of water also helps digestion and absorption of the medication.

2. Take your thyroid hormone medication at the same time each day:

When you take your thyroid medication at the same time each day, this helps your hormone levels remain more stable than if you take it at different times each day. Most thyroid medications have a long half-life of several days. However, even very small changes in the rhythm of your dosage can affect the way you feel. According to the manufacturers of thyroid medications, the hormone will peak in the body at a certain time after ingesting it and then remain stable for a period and afterward have a slightly lowered effect. A patient will want to see the peak and stable effects during the day and the lowered effect toward the end of the day, as time for rest and sleep arrives after a day of activities.

3. If you take vitamins or supplements containing iron or calcium, be sure to take them six hours apart from your thyroid medication dose:

These two supplements can have a negative effect on thyroid hormone medication, by preventing it from fully absorbing in the body. To prevent malabsorption, it is recommended that you take these supplements at least six hours apart from your thyroid medication each day. Some patients will take their thyroid medication in the morning on an empty stomach and then will take their supplements containing iron and/or calcium after lunch, six hours later, to prevent this problem.

4. When you have blood retests of your thyroid hormone levels, take your medication at the same time, to correlate with each blood draw:

Some patients on the day of a blood draw (to retest their thyroid hormone levels) will skip their thyroid medication dose until after their blood is drawn. Other patients will take their thyroid medication dose before the blood draw but will make sure the blood is drawn at the same time for each retest, to make sure levels are consistent in correlation with it. It really is not that important which method you use, if you do so consistently for each blood draw to retest your thyroid hormone levels while being treated for hypothyroidism.

5. Never adjust your own thyroid medication dose:

There can be times when symptoms may manifest themselves even though you took your thyroid medication. This might make some patients believe that a slight increase in their dose that day would help relieve these symptoms, and consequently they are tempted to take it upon themselves to increase their dose. This is never a good idea, without the consent and supervision of your doctor; even small adjustments in your dose can alter your hormone levels for days at a time. If a patient seems to be experiencing symptoms of low thyroid hormone or those of an overactive thyroid (too much hormone), they should report these to their doctor for instructions on adjusting their medication or in making an office visit for further evaluation of their treatment.

6. Hyperthyroidism and Its Causes

Hyperthyroidism is a term simply meaning that one has an "overactive thyroid gland". The metabolism of a person with hyperthyroidism is sped-up from too much thyroid hormone in their system, so that everything in the body is running at overdrive. When this happens, the person will experience hyperthyroid symptoms which include: rapid heart rate, hyperventilation, hypertension, sweating, inability to sleep, nervousness and anxiety, diarrhea, excessive energy followed by fatigue, hair loss, weight loss and swelling of the thyroid gland (a "toxic diffuse goiter" -- which can be painful).

Most people with hyperthyroidism (95%) have Grave's Disease as the cause. This is an autoimmune disease caused by antibodies created by the immune system, that attach to the thyroid gland and stimulate it to produce excessive amounts of hormones. The main antibodies responsible for causing Grave's Disease are called "Thyroid Stimulating Immunoglobulins" (TSI). When a person has hyperthyroidism, these antibodies are blood-tested for, to determine whether the cause is from this common autoimmune thyroid disease.

Most people with Grave's Disease have "toxic diffuse goiters", meaning they have an enlarged thyroid that is over-producing. These type goiters are also commonly painful in newly diagnosed Grave's patients. This disease can also present with complications and co-morbid conditions, including one called "Thyroid Eye Disease" (TED) -- an inflammatory condition that can cause swelling and bulging of the eyes and possible loss of vision, if not treated early.

Another cause of hyperthyroidism are tumors called "thyroid nodules" that can develop in a person's thyroid gland. These will begin to absorb iodine and produce thyroid hormones, as if they have become a part of the thyroid gland. These types are called "hot nodules" and they are a less-common cause of hyperthyroidism. When these types of nodules do cause thyroid hormone imbalance, it is sometimes referred to as "nodular thyroid disease". Rarely, in some women, tumors on their ovaries can also cause hyperthyroidism as can tumors that occur rarely within the pituitary gland.

While Grave's Disease is considered a type of autoimmune thyroiditis, there are non-autoimmune types of temporary thyroiditis that can also cause periods of hyperthyroidism, before they resolve over several weeks or months. The most common type of temporary thyroiditis causing hyperthyroidism, is called "sub-acute thyroiditis".

Lastly, there are medications containing high levels of iodine that can result in the patient taking them, to experience hyperthyroidism. The same is true of iodine found in over-the-counter supplements and in products containing high levels of iodized salt.

If you experience some or all the symptoms listed in the first paragraph of this article, see your doctor about being tested for hyperthyroidism. The most common blood test ordered to detect over-activity by the thyroid gland is the "TSH" (pituitary hormone that reflects thyroid hormone levels). Some doctors will also order tests of the "T4 and T3" thyroid hormone levels if the TSH level is abnormally low (it decreases with too much thyroid hormone). If thyroid hormones are found to be high, tests for Grave's Disease (including TSI antibodies) would likely follow.

7. Treatments for Graves' Disease - Hyperthyroidism

Graves' disease is an autoimmune thyroid disorder that requires treatment by medical professionals. The disease causes the thyroid gland to produce excessive amounts of hormone, causing an over-active metabolism.

With Graves' disease (GD) causing an overactive thyroid gland (hyperthyroidism), the purpose of treatment is to bring thyroid function back to a normal level. An overactive thyroid gland resulting from GD causes too much thyroid hormone to be produced and distributed throughout the body. This will result in an overactive metabolism and in all bodily functions being abnormally sped up. The goal of treatment for GD is to reduce the over-activity of the thyroid gland, so that it is operating at a range considered to be within normal limits. Some of the more common symptoms of GD-hyperthyroidism, are anxiety and nervousness, excessive sweating, rapid heartbeat, hyperventilating, diarrhea and rapid weight loss.

Anti-thyroid medications are used to slow production of thyroid hormones. The thyroid gland produces mainly the "T-4 and T-3" hormones, but people with GD will have increased production of these as a result of the autoimmune response within the body that causes the disease (due mainly to elevated "TSI Antibodies"). Patients will be given a trial of an anti-thyroid medication, which is designed to slow down the overactive thyroid so that thyroid hormones fall within normal values. Two of the more common brands of anti-thyroid medications are methimazole (Tapazole) and propylthiouracil (PTU).

Beta-blocker medications may also be used to control some of the symptoms of hyperthyroidism caused by GD. Beta-blockers, commonly prescribed for high blood pressure, are drugs that partially block the effects of adrenaline, which is the hormone sent out by the adrenal gland that helps stimulate heart rate and blood pressure regulation. Patients with GD may have increased heart rate (tachycardia) and increased blood pressure (hypertension), so administration of a beta-blocker as part of their treatment regimen may sometimes be used to control these abnormally high functioning bodily responses. Some GD patients may only be treated with a beta-blocker or only with an anti-thyroid medication, while some may be treated with both medications simultaneously.

Patients who have GD that cannot be controlled well using oral medications may need their thyroid gland surgically removed or destroyed through radiation treatment (via Radioactive Iodine dosing). The names for thyroid-removal surgeries are "Total Thyroidectomy" (entire gland removal) and "Subtotal Thyroidectomy" (partial gland removal). Once surgery has been performed, there is less or none of the thyroid gland in the patient's body to over-produce thyroid hormones. The same is true of radioactive iodine treatment (also called "RAI ablation"), which is used to destroy the thyroid gland, rather than removing it surgically. Patients afterward have no thyroid gland in their bodies and so become hypothyroid (low thyroid hormone) following removal or ablation. With both types of thyroid removal treatments, the patient will have to be replaced lifelong with the missing hormone, through "Thyroid Hormone Replacement Therapy" (daily medication).

When GD patients develop "Graves' Ophthalmopathy" (GO), this will also need to be treated. This condition, also called "Thyroid Eye Disease" (TED) is a co-occurring inflammatory condition affecting the eyes. It can potentially develop in GD patients and can cause bulging of the eyes and possible deterioration of vision.

The most common treatments for GO include:

*Eye drops to keep the eyes lubricated

*Corticosteroid therapy (oral steroid anti-inflammatory drugs)

*Radiotherapy and/or Decompression Therapy to reduce orbital damage

*Eyelid surgery, to lengthen eyelids that may not cover the eyes well, due to them bulging.

GD patients who smoke are sometimes also advised by their doctors to quit smoking because of the inflammatory chemicals contained in cigarettes that can potentially affect the eyes.

These are general overviews of some more common treatments for GD and GO. Patients with the disease are evaluated by licensed physicians, so that the treatment is tailored to each of them individually.

8. Hypothyroid and Hyperthyroid Simultaneously

An unusual condition can occur in patients with Hashimoto's thyroiditis, in which they phase between being hypothyroid and hyperthyroid. This thyroid disease phenomenon is called "Hashitoxicosis".

While many hypothyroid patients who live in the industrialized countries of the world are not aware of this fact, the cause of their thyroid hormone imbalance is most likely "Hashimoto's thyroiditis".

Some Hashimoto's Hypothyroid Patients Experience 'Hashitoxicosis'

While Hashimoto's typically causes hypothyroidism (low thyroid hormone levels) some patients can have fluctuations in their thyroid hormones, that go from hypothyroid to hyperthyroid (from abnormally-low to abnormally-high thyroid hormones) and this can be due to them having high levels of a certain type of thyroid antibody. The condition I refer to is "Hashitoxicosis". The antibodies that are blood tested for, when Hashimoto's is being determined/diagnosed, are the anti-TPO (anti-thyroid peroxidase) and the anti-TG (anti-thyroglobulin) antibodies (also referred to as "autoantibodies"). Either or both testing positive helps to confirm presence of this hypothyroid disease.

However, some Hashimoto's patients can also test positive for autoimmunity cells called the "TSI" antibodies (Thyroid Stimulating Immunoglobulin). This antibody is what usually contributes to Grave's

Disease or "autoimmune hyperthyroidism" however, some Hashimoto's patients have these antibodies at high levels, as well as having the TPO and/or TG ones, that typically cause Hashimoto's. Therefore, they may experience spells of Hashitoxicosis or "intermittent hyperthyroidism". You could almost say they are suffering from Grave's and Hashimoto's, simultaneously, usually for a limited period of time. This phenomenon is most prominent during the early stage of Hashimoto's and for many patients, the hyperthyroid phases will diminish over time.

With Hashitoxicosis, Symptoms of Hypothyroidism Alternate with Hyperthyroidism

Following, is a list showing the some of the opposite symptoms of hypothyroidism and hyperthyroidism, that Hashimoto's patients can experience in an alternating fashion, when Hashitoxicosis is present.

- constipation alternating with diarrhea
- fatigue alternating with high energy levels
- feeling cold alternating with feeling hot
- having bodily dryness alternating with excessive sweating
- gaining weight alternating with rapid weight loss
- a constant need to sleep alternating with insomnia
- depressed mood alternating with anxiety and nervousness
- slowed heart rate alternating with rapid heart rate
- lack of libido alternating with increased sex drive
- slowed respiration alternating with hyperventilation

'Block and Replace' Treatment for Non-Resolving Hashitoxicosis

Even without having the TSI antibodies present, Hashimoto's patients can potentially experience flares of thyroiditis, which can also cause mild hyperthyroid type symptoms that are not as severe as those caused by Hashitoxicosis but that are still concerning. Doctors will only recognize Hashitoxicosis, if phases of hyperthyroidism symptoms are severe. Some patients who have both Hashimoto's and Grave's antibodies that cause continually unstable thyroid hormone levels and that does not resolve over time, are sometimes placed on a treatment called "block and replace".

This is a treatment in which they will block the hyper-stimulation of the thyroid with an anti-thyroid drug (the medication slows hormone production) and afterward, at the appropriate timing, they will give the patient thyroid hormone therapy (replacing the diminished thyroid hormone levels).This is an alternative treatment to thyroid removal (thyroidectomy and ablation), however, if the treatment fails, once given an ample trial, thyroid removal might be recommended as a follow up treatment.

Block and Replace Test Trials

According to medical research studies published by the U.S.-NIH (PubMed website), the Block and Replace treatment has also been administered to Graves' disease patients, who phase between being euthyroid (normal thyroid hormone levels) and having overt hyperthyroidism. These patients are not experiencing Hashitoxcosis, in which their thyroid hormone levels drop to hypothyroid levels naturally (without treatment influence).

The trials have had varied rates of success in providing test patients with periods of Graves' disease remission. In recent years the treatment has been administered to patients, during test trails in the UK. Click on this article-title, to read a research article abstract on the subject: "Treatment of Graves' disease with the block-replace regimen of antithyroid drugs: the effect of treatment duration and immunogenetic susceptibility on relapse."

For Most Hashimoto's Patients – Hashitoxicosis Resolves on Its Own

Some Hashimoto's patients have been known to transition over to Grave's Disease over time, when having both types of antibodies (those that destroy thyroid cells and those that stimulate thyroid hormone production) and they become progressively hyperthyroid (not common). Most Hashimoto's patients who experience Hashitoxicosis however, will have intermittent hyperthyroid phases for a period of weeks or months but they will still become progressively hypothyroid afterward and there comes a point at which the Hashitoxicosis resolves and never returns.

It should be encouraging for patients who experience Hashitoxicosis to know that many Hashimoto's patients, only have the hyperthyroid spells more-so during the early onset of their disease but with time, the hyperthyroidism phases subside and give way to progressive hypothyroidism, which is easily-treated with a daily dose of thyroid hormone replacement medication.

9. Thyroid Hormones and Antibodies

Following are two general, common questions asked by thyroid patients (QUESTION ONE has 2 parts), with my researched answers following each of them.

QUESTION ONE (Part 1): I'm taking thyroid hormone replacement but also taking a thyroid extract supplement, what do you think about this combination?

ANSWER: To be honest, I'm wary of thyroid extract supplements because they sometimes vary in dose-to-dose consistency and when added to your prescription thyroid hormone, have the potential to over-dose you and cause hyperthyroid symptoms (thyro-toxicity). I'm a stickler for prescribed thyroid hormone (they are USP and/or FDA approved), that is monitored by a treating doctor.

QUESTION ONE (Part 2): This combination regimen is already being administered and monitored by my treating doctor does this make it a safer option?

ANSWER: If your doctor is over-seeing your regimen of both, that is a whole different story and as long as he is retesting your blood levels, I would think it might work great for you.

Also the "thyroid extract" may be a specific type supplement that contains an exact amount of T3 and/or T4 in it and may be referred-to as an extract in certain parts of the U.S. or other countries but is actually a high quality supplement closely-regulated. It might even have the USP approval on it. I mention this because there are two Canadian brands called Nature Thyroid and Westthroid (possibly discontinued) and while they are sometimes referred-to as thyroid extracts, they are high quality and require a prescription if purchased within the USA. Your Dr. may be a

Naturopath or Holistic doctor but this makes no difference as long as he is good at treating hypothyroidism and retests your blood thyroid hormone levels to monitor your treatment every 6 to 8 weeks until you are well stabilized on your regimen (afterward, testing may only need done 2 or 3 times yearly).

QUESTION: Have you been seeing information on the fact that patients with hypothyroidism caused by Hashimoto's thyroiditis, can have antibodies directed against their TSH receptors which can cause their TSH level to be unreliable when blood-tested to monitor their hypothyroidism?

ANSWER: Yes, I've been seeing more info regarding how common different types of antibodies are in Hashimoto's patients that block TSH (Thyroid Stimulating Hormone) and its receptors which can make their TSH lab results less reliable. Some Hashimoto's patients for example, test positive for the TSI antibodies, that typically cause Graves' disease, and this can cause them transient/temporary phases of hyperthyroidism ("Hashitoxicosis"). This is another reason TSH-only testing is not always a good way to go with diagnosing and for follow-up retests after new patients are started on thyroid hormone replacement therapy (T-4 and T-3 tests should also be included).

I've also been seeing articles and books mentioning that there can also be antibodies present in Hashimoto's patients, directed especially against T-3 specifically. If this proves to be true, this may be why patients on brands of thyroid hormone like Armour (brand I take) have success for a while on the medication and afterward lose some of that improvement because some of the hormone is being destroyed by these antibodies. You would think that simply a dose-increase would over-ride this problem, but I suppose it might not work if the antibodies increased to very high levels. I'll keep watch on these subjects and cover them as we go along. It remains an interesting field of study as they continue to research and find new info and improved treatments!

10. Treating Mixed Thyroid Disease

Some thyroid patients are difficult to regulate on doses of thyroid replacement hormone, as treatment for their hypothyroidism because they shift easily into hyperthyroid states. These patients are sometimes referred for thyroidectomy surgeries (thyroid gland removal) or RAI ablation (destruction of the gland by radioactive iodine). These treatments are rare for hypothyroid patients and thyroid removal is usually only done for hyperthyroid patients who have Graves' disease or for patients who have thyroid nodules (tumors) or goiters, that are causing them problems or that contain malignant cells (cancer).

In my sincere lay-opinion, I feel that hypothyroid patients who experience alternating symptoms between hyperthyroid and hypothyroid, should ask their doctors to order "thyroid antibodies tests". It would be important to make sure the blood panel includes a test to detect "TSI antibodies" ("Thyroid Stimulating Immunoglobulin" -- that typically causes Graves's-hyperthyroidism).

If a hypothyroid patient is having these mixed symptoms, they will likely test positive for the main antibodies that are typically found positive in both Hashimoto's and Graves', which are called the "Anti-TPO" "Anti-TG". However, if they also test positive for TSI, they might be diagnosed with "Hashitoxicosis" (transient hyperthyroidism) or co-occurring Graves' disease (a permanent condition that will continue to cause them hyperthyroid phases).

As far as typical hypothyroid therapy goes, it's not unusual for it to take several trials of thyroid hormone doses in newly treated hypothyroid patients, for their doctors to see what works best for them over time. This is also why it's important to have a doctor who takes real interest in getting the treatment as adequate or optimized as possible.

If over a significant trial-period of time, a patient's levels still fluctuate-widely even while they're on a set dose of hormone, their case may require another qualified Endocrinologist or thyroid specializing doctor for a "second opinion" (to see if a mixed autoimmune condition exists). I always suggest this as simply fellow-patient opinion, especially if thyroidectomy or RAI ablation is recommended, due to a failure of initial thyroid hormone therapy.

Doctors usually only recommend these as last resorts for hypothyroid patients. They are serious procedures and patients should be thoroughly informed about them (e.g. how they are administered and what to expect following them). This would be important, if their doctors are thoroughly convinced that either of them needs to be administered.

Some autoimmune hypothyroid patients who have a rough start on hormone replacement therapy, end up leveling-out fine later; even those who experience an initial time of phasing between hypothyroid and hyperthyroid. The right brand and dose of replacement hormone therapy can also make a difference in lending-toward successful treatment, that doesn't require additional procedures.

11. My Review for - Hypothyroidism Type 2: The Epidemic

Are some cases of hypothyroidism not diagnose-able via the most common method, being that of blood testing? Dr. Mark Starr certainly believes so and he shares those beliefs in this remarkable book.

Dr. Mark Starr's book was a fascinating read for me because I have always felt that among the estimated 13 million people suffering from thyroid disease -- that remain undiagnosed, many of them have cases of hypothyroidism, that are not being detected for lack of proper observational testing -- apart from conventional blood tests.

The Typical Symptoms of Hypothyroidism

The symptoms commonly listed for hypothyroidism, are those that will be experienced by patients with Hypothyroidism Type 2, which may include the following.

- fatigue and malaise

- weight gain

- joint and muscle aches

- depression and/or anxiety

- constipation and slowed digestion

- dry, flaky skin

- slowed heart rate and respiration

- feeling cold in warm climates and low body temperature

- difficulty concentrating (brain fog)

- dry, brittle hair that falls out

- swelling of the face and extremities (edema/myxedema)

When a patient visits their doctor with these types of symptoms, one of the suspected causes would be hypothyroidism. The problem that can arise in regard to Hypothyroidism Type 2, is that a blood test evaluation of the patient, will not reveal the underlying hypothyroid state, that has yet to cause thyroid hormone levels to fall below normal values. The patient will be experiencing full-fledged symptoms of an underactive thyroid gland but their blood lab test results, will be normal.

In these cases, further tests should be done, as discussed in Dr. Starr's book, which would include gauging the patient's "Basal Metabolic Rate" (oxygen consumption within a certain time limit). This would also include taking their "Basal Body Temperature", through a series of readings, via placing a basal thermometer under their arm, first thing in the morning (upon them waking), for several days consecutively. Lastly, this would include performing a close physical examination of the patient, for subtle signs of myxedema – meaning areas of tissue-swelling on/within the patient's body.

Doctors who are familiar with these testing methods, as outlined by Dr. Starr, will sometimes conclude a diagnosis of hypothyroidism in a patient, in spite of all thyroid panel blood tests, falling within normal values

Some in the Medical Community May Disagree

When I saw the title "Hypothyroidism Type 2", it was at first puzzling because I had not heard this term previously. As I ventured deeper into the book, it became clear as to what this term actually meant, and it began to make a great deal of sense to me. I'm sure Dr. Starr is aware of the fact and has likely already experienced the fact, that there is opposition out there in the medical community, in recognizing hypothyroidism that is not detectable and diagnose-able through blood lab testing alone. This book brings recognition to just such a disease, that causes the same symptoms as blood lab-detectable hypothyroidism (Type 1).

The over 250 page book which I was provided a free copy of from Dr. Starr, sheds much light on the fact that this blood lab elusive type of thyroid hormone dysfunction has as its origin, genetic inheritance of inadequate thyroid hormone metabolism (faulty genes) and environmental toxins, both of which have been passed down through the generations, with increasing incidence of Hypothyroidism Type 2. It seems highly evident that this type of underactive thyroid gland, does in fact affect a significant percent of the general population, in spite of any disagreements that might arise within the medical community, to the contrary.

Observations for Hypothyroidism Before Availability of Blood Testing

Dr. Starr, who is Board Certified in pain medicine gives extremely convincing documentation for this disease which had its recognition, even before the development of thyroid function blood testing. The pioneering medical researchers who studied hypothyroidism, during its earliest recognition, as detailed in this book, had no choice but to diagnose hypothyroidism based upon the patient's signs and symptoms and by use of physical diagnostic methods that may in reality, still be better indicators of the more subtle forms of hypothyroidism. Thyroid blood testing was not yet available at that time.

The early tests used in the pioneering days of diagnosing hypothyroidism that Dr. Starr talks about in his book, include tests of patient's Basal Metabolic Rates, in which a patient's oxygen consumption was measured and their Basal Temperatures were measured (metabolic body temperature). These early diagnoses of patients also included observation for the presence of "myxedema", which presents as marked puffiness and swelling of bodily tissues, which was also an early term for hypothyroidism.

Proof that these types of tests and observations were often accurate in diagnosing hypothyroidism was the fact that when these patients were treated with thyroid hormone replacement therapy, they improved remarkably. Many photos and symptom-charts are included in the book, showing these patient's before and after their improvements, from a time-period before diagnostic blood testing was available.

Hypothyroid Disease Research Continues

Dr. Starr has dedicated many years of research to this disease, studying the research of the pioneers of Endocrinology, in addition to conducting his own test-research. These fathers of thyroid research include the renowned British MD – Dr. Ord, who first identified various types of thyroid disease including autoimmune thyroiditis. Dr. Broda O. Barnes is also included among these pioneers, who also has a research foundation named after him, that continues his work to this day. Dr. Starr has also studied directly with Dr. Hans Kraus -- a professor of the Rusk Institute (now deceased), who was one of the doctors who treated President John F. Kennedy's Addison's' Disease and hypothyroidism.

There is in fact, also a foreword for the book, written by Dr. Thomas D. Broc, B.Sc., D.D.S., who has been successfully treated for Hypothyroidism Type 2 by Dr. Starr. In the foreword this doctor points out the fact that he could not be diagnosed previously, due to thyroid function blood labs not detecting his hypothyroidism. Dr. Starr himself has also experienced relief from a pain condition he suffered as well, due to this type of hypothyroidism, once he received thyroid hormone replacement therapy.

The cited studies and documentation in this book for Hypothyroidism Type 2 are extensive and include studies from autopsies, examination of umbilical cords and the presence of toxic chemicals and pollutants in the environment, that adversely affect thyroid function. The book also provides a better understanding of the function of thyroid hormones, in aiding "mitochondria" (energy producing cells), in regulating the body's metabolism and how this process can be hindered through genetic predisposition and environmental toxins/pollutants.

This Reader is Convinced

I have barely scratched the surface in describing the information contained in this book and so I will simply sum up my experience in reading it, by saying that it is extremely well-documented and provides more-than-ample proof for each point that is made in regard to the illness Dr. Starr has amply-named "Hypothyroidism Type 2". I highly recommend the book to readers who enjoy resources on highly interesting thyroid disease subjects.

SECTION TWO

Testing for Thyroid Disorders

TABLE OF CONTENTS:

5. Incredible Sensitivity of TSH Blood Testing

6. Nutritional Deficiencies and Hypothyroid Therapy

7. Symptoms that Merit Thyroid Blood Tests

8. Taking Thyroid Medication Before a Blood Draw

9. Thyroid Autoimmunity and Temporary Thyroiditis

10. Thyroid Disease a Risk for Related Conditions

11. Treating Thyroid Hormone Conversion Failure

12. TSH Blood Test Considerations

13. My Review For: The Thyroid Diet Revolution

1. Basics about Thyroid Function Tests

Blood testing is the most common, initial method of evaluating thyroid hormone levels, to determine if hyperthyroidism or hypothyroidism is present. Afterward, thyroid imaging scans might follow.

Blood tests are the most used medical method, for diagnosing thyroid diseases and hormone imbalances.

Thyroid Imaging Tests

Occasionally doctors use additional tests when needed, including one called an "Iodine Uptake Scan". This test of thyroid function uses radioactive iodine, given to a patient in a small dose, followed by radiological imaging, that is done once the thyroid gland absorbs/uptakes the iodine. With this test a doctor can determine at what percent the thyroid is functioning properly and if any areas of the gland are failing. Normal values for the "6-hour test" are 3% to 16% and for the "24-hour test", normal values are 8% to 25%.

The Uptake Scan can also detect the presence of thyroid nodules (tumorous growths) and helps determine the types they are (e.g. stimulating or non-stimulating to the thyroid gland). A "Thyroid Ultrasound" is similar but images are made by means of highly sensitive sound waves. While this test does not determine how well the thyroid is functioning, it can reveal when there are any nodules present within the gland, goiters (swelling) and abnormal thyroid tissue (e.g. diseased or cancerous areas on or within the gland).

Thyroid Blood Panels

The more common tests from blood draw samples, are in groupings called "Thyroid Panels" or each test may be done separately. A thyroid panel, will include what most doctors agree to be the most diagnostic and sensitive test, called "TSH" (Thyroid Stimulating Hormone). This hormone, being an indicator of thyroid function, does not come from the thyroid gland itself but rather from a gland found in the brain, called the "pituitary".

This master brain-gland regulates many of the body's endocrine hormones and TSH is the hormone it sends to the thyroid gland, to regulate its production of the actual thyroid hormones, the major ones being the "T-3 and T-4". These are the two major hormones that the thyroid gland itself, disperses-out for regulating bodily-metabolism, in response to being stimulated by TSH to do so. The T-3 and T-4 hormones are made up of iodine molecules, T-3 having three iodine molecules and T-4 having four iodine molecules. The TSH level in the blood and also the thyroid hormones T-3 and T-4 are the ones that can best-determine how the thyroid is functioning and these are the three that are most often combined on a thyroid function blood panel.

Recent Changes in TSH Normal Values for Blood Testing Labs

In the year 2002, the "AACE" (American Association of Clinical Endocrinologists), revised the standard for TSH testing. The "normal range" was changed due to their ongoing medical research studies, which concluded that the old TSH range was too broad. As a result, they narrowed it, so that more patients with developing thyroid disease, could be diagnosed earlier. The old TSH range was generally "0.5 to 5.0", with the revised range being roughly "0.3 to 3.0". Some blood testing labs are still using the older reference range, while many have adjusted theirs to

meet the new guidelines.

When a patient is tested for TSH, they need to have a result from the blood sample that fits within the reference range, to be considered normal. If they have a reading below 0.3, this would possibly indicate hyper-functioning (hyperthyroidism) of the thyroid gland because this means the pituitary is backing-off from sending more TSH, after it senses that too much thyroid hormone, is already being released by the thyroid gland. On the other hand, if a patient's blood result is above 3.0, this possibly indicates hypo-functioning of the thyroid gland (hypothyroidism) because not enough thyroid hormones are being made to lower the TSH, which makes it remain abnormally high.

Various Versions of Thyroid Function Panels

The T-4 and T-3 blood tests come in a variety of different versions, such as the "totals" of each or the "free" levels of each, or they are combined in tests called the "FTI Index" and the "T-7". There is also one called the "T-3 Uptake" but this one actually measures how well the thyroid gland "uptakes" and utilizes the T-3 hormone, via the available globulins found in the bloodstream (a diseased thyroid uptakes less T-3). All these tests help to determine thyroid function and hormone production levels and all of them have lab ranges with a "below-normal" result indicating hypothyroidism and an "above-normal" result indicating hyperthyroidism (opposite of what TSH does).

Many doctors believe the "TSH", and the "Free T-3 and T-4" are the three best blood tests of thyroid function and these are what they will often place on a thyroid panel. Abnormal readings on any of these, would also likely result in a doctor ordering tests for "thyroid antibodies" (cells from the immune system that attack the thyroid), to determine if any thyroid dysfunction is due to autoimmune disease of the thyroid gland (the most common cause in industrialized countries of the world).

As it stands today, blood tests are recognized as the most superior, initial method for determining how well a patent's thyroid gland is functioning.

2. Can TSH Blood Testing Be Inaccurate?

The TSH blood test is extremely valuable for diagnosing and treating thyroid disease patients but in a small percent of cases, it is not accurate in reflecting the T3 and/or T4 thyroid hormone levels.

TSH or "Thyroid Stimulating Hormone", is the pituitary gland hormone that regulates thyroid function and when levels of it are blood-tested, it is an extremely sensitive and highly diagnostic thyroid function indicator, in most cases. It is especially valuable in diagnosing developing thyroid hormone imbalances, earlier than any other blood thyroid function test. With this said, it should always be understood that there are some cases in which TSH does not accurately reflect the thyroid hormone levels of some patients. Therefore, in the opinion of some thyroid specializing MDs, doctors should order more than "TSH alone", when diagnosing thyroid diseases but also when monitoring the thyroid hormone replacement therapy, of treated hypothyroid patients. A complete thyroid panel that also includes the T-4 and T-3 levels, can ensure against failed diagnoses of thyroid hormone imbalances and inadequately treated hypothyroid patients.

Obvious Reasons TSH Can Be Inaccurate

There are some obvious reasons why TSH is not an accurate reflection of thyroid hormone levels (of the T-4 and T-3), such as when hypothyroidism is caused by a problem within the pituitary gland (where TSH comes from), which is referred to a "Central Hypothyroidism" -- meaning an underactive thyroid gland is originating from the brain center. This type would also be in the "Secondary Hypothyroidism" category -- meaning it is caused by something other than the thyroid gland itself. There are also syndromes referred to as "Low T-3 Syndrome" and "Euthyroid Sick Syndrome", which are caused by other illnesses that are occurring in the body, rather than from a diseased or damaged thyroid gland and that result in a low T-3 level, while T-4 and TSH remain within normal range, at the same time. Diseases such as Juvenile Diabetes and a stress related illness called "Wilson's Temperature Syndrome" can be a cause of low T-3 levels as well, with T-4 and TSH seemingly unaffected. In these cases, a test of the "TSH only" or even a combination of "TSH and T-4", would not detect these low T-3 syndromes.

Rare Causes of Inaccuracies in Thyroid Stimulating Hormone

Other causes of an inaccurate TSH level, however, are not typical and sometimes there is no clear explanation as to why TSH does not accurately reflect the thyroid hormone levels in some patients. I the author of this Hub, have seen the testimonials of patients who had thyroid hormone levels that were at hypothyroid level but their TSH was in the normal range. When their pituitary function was also tested, to see if that was the problem, test results indicated normal pituitary function. In these cases, there was no explanation for why TSH and the thyroid hormones were not correlating as they should. It is possible that any abnormal pituitary function in these patients, sub-clinical (mild hypopituitarism) and not showing up on pituitary function testing. It could also be that these patients have other hormone imbalances such as low adrenal or sex hormones, affecting the endocrine system (all glands that produce hormones) and causing a problem in communication between the pituitary and thyroid glands.

Mildly Low-Functioning Endocrine System

Giving myself for an example, I have an overall mild, general endocrine dysfunction, according to my doctors, that causes me to need a very suppressed TSH level, for my thyroid hormone therapy to be effective in treating my hypothyroidism. Unless my TSH is suppressed "below normal", my thyroid hormone levels will not reach mid-range or above. While cases like mine are not common, they do exist and I have corresponded with several other patients, since my own diagnosis in 2003, who have experienced this same scenario. If my doctor started out testing only my TSH to monitor my thyroid hormone therapy, I would have been under-treated for it, to this very day.

I feel with these possibilities happening to a small percent of patients like myself, it is only good medical common sense, to test patients diagnostically and in follow-up on thyroid hormone therapy, via their levels of TSH, Free T-4 and Free T-3 (a thyroid panel, as opposed to a single test), for at least the first time or two, to make sure TSH correlates with both thyroid hormone levels, in each individual patient.

3. Determining the Cause of Hypothyroidism

There are many causes for an underactive thyroid gland. Some are more common than others, such as "thyroid autoimmunity" (common) and "toxic chemical exposure" (rare). Tests can often reveal causes.

When a person receives a medical diagnosis of hypothyroidism, the next logical question they might ask their doctors would be "why do I have this condition -- what caused me to develop it?"

Some newly diagnosed hypothyroid patients may have doctors who don't believe in filling in any details other than those of most importance. They might answer with a reply to a patient's question regarding the "cause" of their hypothyroidism, to the effective that "it's just one of those things that happens to lots of people". Many patients, however, will want to know what was responsible for their thyroid hormone imbalance, that has reached the point of needing treated for the rest of their lives. Usually, with more investigation, consisting of further blood tests or thyroid imaging tests, a definitive cause for cases of hypothyroidism can be determined.

Causes determined for diagnosed hypothyroid cases, may include the following.

•   Thyroid autoimmunity - immune cells attacking the thyroid gland (diagnosed by tests for thyroid antibodies and thyroid tissue biopsy)

- Malfunctioning brain glands - usually problems with the pituitary or hypothalamus (diagnosed by magnetic resonance imaging "MRI"

- Old age - atrophy/shrinkage of the thyroid gland over time (diagnosed by patient history and thyroid ultrasound imaging)

- Toxic chemical exposure - usually radioactivity (diagnosed by patient's history)

- Following pregnancy - usually temporary until nutrients are replaced (diagnosed by blood tests and patient history)

- Following birth - usually temporary until an infant's thyroid strengthens (diagnosed by Newborn Screening blood tests)

- Low T3 syndromes - usually temporary, from severe, chronic stress or other diseases (diagnosed by thyroid blood panel that includes the "T3" hormone level)

- Thyroid cancer - healthy thyroid tissue is replaced by abnormal malignant tissue (diagnosed by thyroid tissue biopsy)

Some cases of hypothyroidism have obvious causes as some of the factors in the preceding list reveals, while others are more elusive. I will now mention some cases that may require thorough investigation to determine the causes of them

According to medical research that has been conducted, some cases of Hashimoto's thyroiditis -- the common autoimmune cause of hypothyroidism, do not present with positive antibodies blood tests but will only be detected by Fine Needle Aspiration (thyroid tissue biopsy). An article by one online source that addresses this medical scenario, is titled "Hashimoto's thyroiditis: fine-needle aspirations of 50 asymptomatic cases." (published by the U.S.-NIH "PubMed" website)

While autoimmune thyroiditis is often the cause of progressive hypothyroidism, viral thyroiditis and sub-acute forms usually present with hyperthyroidism (an overactive thyroid), which resolves within a few weeks and are not followed by progressive hypothyroidism. Analysis of a thyroid tissue sample would be differentiated by a reviewing specialist, as to the difference between a transient type of thyroiditis and a permanent, autoimmune type. A test of this type might become necessary if hypothyroidism has been found present in a patient, who also happens to be experiencing viral thyroiditis at the same time. In some cases, it may be found that the thyroiditis and the hypothyroidism are separate issues and that the occurrence of them at the same time, is coincidental. It would be this very type of scenario, in which blood testing alone might not reveal the cause of hypothyroidism but a tissue biopsy would provide a more definitive answer as to the cause.

In regard to other causes of hypothyroidism, supplements that contain high levels of iodine have been shown to contribute to thyroid autoimmunity resulting in either Grave's disease hyperthyroidism or Hashimoto's thyroiditis hypothyroidism, in some people who take them -- according to medical research published by the U.S.-NIH. In a case like this, an investigating doctor would want to question the patient about any supplements they have been taking, that could have possibly resulted in the development of thyroid disease, that led to their case of hypothyroidism.

I, the author, recently heard from a friend of mine, in regard to his development of hypothyroidism after taking an herbal supplement, that he felt triggered in him a case of non-resolving thyroiditis. It is possible (but not certain) that the supplement my friend had been taking was causing him to be hypothyroid and if he had stopped taking it much sooner, it might have corrected his developing thyroid hormone imbalance.

It's difficult to imagine that an over-the-counter supplement would have caused him permanent thyroid damage. However, while it's possible that it did in-fact result from the natural remedy, it could more-specifically be because there was some other toxic agent within the product, that he was unaware of, which caused permanent damage to his thyroid gland. People vary in their tolerance to herbal supplements, so anything is possible (toxins have also been known to show up in products made by unreliable, non-reputable companies).

If the cause of a hypothyroid condition is not within the thyroid gland itself -- "primary", it can be a secondary cause. Since there are many possible causes, including secondary ones, such as other disease processes going on within the body, age-related (if elderly), or thyroid regulating brain gland problems -- "Central Hypothyroidism", it may take considerable testing and a process of elimination to find a definitive cause in these cases as well. Some doctors aren't too concerned about "cause", because they simply treat the under active thyroid and if treatment improves it, they call it good. Most patients do however want to know the cause of their hypothyroidism, if possible (some doctors do as well), so that they know more about what's been going on in their bodies.

In regard to types of hypothyroidism resulting from only one thyroid hormone being low -- namely the T3 level, in my opinion as a layperson - non medical professional, the T4 and T3 hormone levels should be blood-tested to see if only the T3 is lowering in new cases of hypothyroidism that have no obvious cause determined for them. This can happen with "low T3 syndromes" like "Wilson's Temperature Syndrome" and "Euthyroid Sick Syndrome" and occasionally in cardiac patients as well.

I have mentioned the preceding things, which demonstrate the fact that causes for hypothyroidism can be highly varied within certain groups of people, in whom there isn't an obvious cause that manifests. Regardless, most patients want their doctors to zero-in on the cause of their hypothyroidism, so that they can know details about what has given them a lifelong disease, that will require them to be medically-treated, for the rest of their lives.

4. Hereditary Thyroid Disease

Is thyroid disease sometimes passed down from generation to generation? What factor does congenital hyperthyroidism and hypothyroidism play in hereditary thyroid disorders and are they treatable?

A common question people have regarding hereditary thyroid disease would be this: "What are the chances for a child of a thyroid disease parent, to eventually experience the onset of the same disease or to even be born with it?" In searching and researching this subject, I found conclusions and views on the subject, which I will discuss, following. ---

Medical Statistics on Inherited Thyroid Disease

According to Dr. Hossein Gharib, M.D. of the American Association of Clinical Endocrinologists and Professor at the Mayo Medical School, "Fifty percent of thyroid disease patients' offspring will inherit the thyroid disease gene."

Even as a Thyroid Patient Advocate, I didn't know that chances for children of thyroid disease parents were at 50% risk, for also experiencing the disease, until I found the quote from Dr. Gharib -- medical professor. I knew it was a high percent risk but 50% was surprising. That's not great news for children of thyroid disease parents but it shows the importance of getting blood tested at any point thyroid disease symptoms arise and if they don't manifest earlier in life, to start getting tested at age 35. The

American Thyroid Association in fact states that everyone be screened yearly for thyroid disease starting at age 35 and every 5 years thereafter.

I, the author am a rare case, in that there have been no known thyroid disease cases, on either side of my family, even tracing them back several generations. Therefore, I was not tested for thyroid disease and diagnosed with "Hashimoto's thyroiditis" (autoimmune hypothyroidism), until age 40, when I developed symptoms.

Reputable thyroid disease statistics show that ages 35 to 40 are common for people to experience the onset of thyroid disease. If you are the child of a parent or you are a parent with thyroid disease, you should educate yourself about thyroid disease symptoms, so that you can recognize when there might be a need for blood testing.

Following is a list of the most common symptoms experienced by people who have developed hypothyroidism or hyperthyroidism.

Main Symptoms of Hypothyroidism (Underactive Thyroid)

- fatigue
- constipation
- excessive need to sleep
- depression
- dry skin
- slow vital signs (breathing and heart rate)

Main Symptoms of Hyperthyroidism (Overactive Thyroid)

- hyper energy levels

- diarrhea

- insomnia

- anxiety/nervousness

- sweaty/oily skin

- sped-up vital signs

The Need to Test for "Thyroid Antibodies"

When symptoms arise in someone at risk for developing thyroid disease, they should not only have tests ordered for thyroid function but also those that detect "thyroid antibodies". These are killer cells that the immune system creates and sends-out to attack what it perceives to be invaders in the body (e.g. viruses, bacteria and allergens). In the case of autoimmune thyroid disease, it recognizes the thyroid as one of those invaders. These antibodies can cause thyroid disease symptoms in advance of causing eventual thyroid hormone imbalance and this is why they are important tests to order, along with thyroid hormone panels.

Thyroid antibodies tests include the "anti-thyroid peroxidase" (abbreviated "anti-TPO"), the "anti-thyroglobulin" (abbreviated "anti-TG") and "thyroid stimulating immunoglobulin" (abbreviated "TSI"). The first two I mention (anti-TPO and Anti-TG) are common findings and will test positive in autoimmune hypothyroidism or "Hashimoto's thyroiditis", while the third one I listed (TSI), is more commonly found in people with autoimmune hyperthyroidism or "Grave's Disease". So, depending upon the symptoms one is having, they may want only certain antibodies tested for and this should be discussed with their doctors.

Tests Commonly Used to Evaluate Thyroid Function

Thyroid function tests, that detect hormone imbalances, are the "TSH", "T4" and "T3" levels. Some doctors believe the "Free levels" of the T4 and T3 are best. These are the ones that I, the author has tested in follow up on my thyroid hormone therapy for hypothyroidism, but they are also good for diagnosing thyroid disorders. If only one test is used to evaluate thyroid function, it will usually be the "TSH" level (Thyroid Stimulating Hormone). This one is the pituitary hormone that accurately reflects how well the thyroid gland is supplying hormone to the body and is highly sensitive in that it usually detects a change in thyroid function earlier than any other test.

Newborns Screenings for Babies at Risk for Hereditary Thyroid Disease

The term "Congenital Hypothyroidism", is one describing infants born with under-functioning thyroid glands. On the opposite side of the spectrum, would be babies born with "Congenital Hyperthyroidism" but hyperthyroid newborns (those with overactive thyroid glands) are so rare, that there are no published statistics for the occurrence of them, in relationship to the number of newborns delivered each year in general. Hypothyroid newborns, however, are a significant enough occurrence, as to require all newborns to be screened for thyroid hormone imbalances at birth.

Babies born with hypothyroidism, are usually diagnosed when undergoing blood tests called "Newborn Screenings" which are done to determine the immediate health of them. Some babies may display symptoms of being ill with congenital hypothyroidism while others may appear healthy, but their low functioning thyroid is still discovered through blood tests. If symptoms do occur, they will be somewhat different from those experienced by adults and may include the following.

- Constipation or diarrhea
- jaundice (yellowing of the skin)
- lack of appetite
- difficulty breathing
- sleeping more than is normal
- enlargement of the head, tongue or stomach.

More than Heredity Can Be Involved in Newborn Thyroid Disorders

While Congenital Hypothyroidism is not common, its occurrence is found often-enough, that general statistics are showing that it affects an estimated 1 in 3,000 or 4,000 newborns in industrialized countries and is twice as common in girls, than in boys. Estimates are not as easily determined for less-developed countries where blood testing of newborns is not as accessible.

For most infants, a cause of congenital hypothyroidism cannot be determined but in other cases, heredity of the disease may be suspected. Some infants may be affected by medications the mother is taking, including those for an overactive thyroid gland (hyperthyroidism). These type medications are called "anti-thyroid drugs", designed to slow production of thyroid hormones in the mother but may also slow thyroid hormone production in their newborns. Babies born prematurely are also at higher risk for congenital hypothyroidism.

Treatment for Congenital Hypothyroidism Must Begin Immediately

It is important for newborns to begin treatment for congenital hypothyroidism with thyroid hormone replacement therapy because a delay in treating it can cause a slowing of their physical and mental development. The risks of delayed treatment include mental retardation and physical defects involving the muscles, bones and teeth. This points to the great importance in newborn blood screenings because delay in treatment can result in permanent damage to babies at a critical time following their birth.

Some newborns will recover from congenital hypothyroidism, after short term treatment and their own thyroid glands will begin to function normally afterward. Other newborns may require long-term or lifelong treatment, especially those who are born with damaged, underdeveloped or missing thyroid glands.

Adult Diagnosed Cases Will Require Lifetime Treatments

Regarding adults who inherit thyroid disease that is found after age 18, treatment for them will be lifelong in basically all cases. With inherited hypothyroidism, hormone replacement must be continued for the remaining lifetime of the patient and it must be administered lifelong following thyroid removal in cases of hyperthyroidism as well (after thyroidectomy or radioactive iodine ablation of their thyroid gland). If an adult has a case of hyperthyroidism that doesn't require thyroid removal, they will require anti-thyroid drugs and/or beta-blocker medications for their remaining lifetimes as well.

For both congenital and adult cases of thyroid disease that are diagnosed within a proper timing, treatments can restore to them, a relatively normal quality of life.

5. Incredible Sensitivity of TSH Blood Testing

The highly accurate "Thyroid Stimulating Hormone" blood test (TSH), is the one most used to first evaluate a patient's thyroid function for the presence of hypothyroidism or hyperthyroidism.

The "Thyroid Stimulating Hormone" (TSH), does not come from the thyroid gland but rather comes from a major endocrine gland in the brain, called the "pituitary".

Blood TSH Levels Change with Thyroid Hormone Status

Even with TSH not being a thyroid hormone, it still provides an accurate measure (reflection) of thyroid gland function, when levels of it are blood tested. This is because the actions of this hormone, reflect how thyroid function is going in a person's body. It does this, by being sent-out from the pituitary gland in lower amounts when there is already enough thyroid hormone being dispersed into the body and by being sent-out in higher amounts when more thyroid hormones are needed in the body. In people who do not have thyroid disease, this will occur throughout each day, within normal limits. In other words, TSH will fluctuate upward and downward, constantly throughout each 24 hour day but it will do so within the normal values range in people without thyroid hormone imbalances, which is an average of about "0.3 to 4.0", at blood testing labs. Values below 0.3 on blood lab test results, may indicate that a hyperthyroid condition is present (overactive thyroid) and values above 4.0, may indicate that a hypothyroid condition is present (underactive thyroid).

Most Types of Hypothyroidism Cause TSH to Elevate

TSH will begin to fall outside of the normal values range on the low end, when one or both of the main thyroid hormones called T4 and T3, become imbalanced in a person's body due to a thyroid disease/disorder or from a secondary cause that indirectly affects the thyroid gland. With hypothyroidism -- an underactive thyroid for example, TSH will begin to elevate to above normal values because the body of an affected person, is in need of more T4 and/or T3 hormone, to keep their metabolism running properly (the rate at which energy is burned from things consumed). The need for more of these hormones, occurs because the thyroid gland is falling behind in dispersing its own hormones, after becoming damaged, diseased or hindered in some way. The most common disease-causing hypothyroidism is called "Hashimoto's thyroiditis", which is autoimmune destruction of the thyroid gland by cells called "thyroid antibodies".

TSH Does Not Elevate with Central Hypothyroidism

Other non-disease causes of hypothyroid conditions can also occur however, including one called "Central Hypothyroidism" and this type occurs because of a problem within the pituitary gland itself, causing it not to send out enough TSH to stimulate adequate thyroid hormone production. This is usually due to a benign tumor in the pituitary and in this case, the TSH blood-tested level will not show hypothyroidism (TSH will remain low) and it will instead have to be diagnosed by testing the blood levels of T4 and T3 directly. When it is considered how common cases of hypothyroidism are, that are caused by thyroid glands that become diseased, Central Hypothyroidism is rare in comparison.

The TSH Level will Drop to Abnormally Low Levels in Cases of Hyperthyroidism

With hyperthyroidism -- an overactive thyroid, the opposite will occur and TSH will become suppressed, dropping down to below normal values because abnormally high amounts of thyroid hormones are already being produced, causing a sped-up metabolism in the affected person's body. Hyperthyroidism is also usually caused by a diseased thyroid gland and the two main diseases that can cause it, are "Graves' disease" and small tumorous growths that can develop within the gland, called "hot nodules".

With Graves' disease, thyroid antibody destruction of the gland occurs, like in Hashimoto's thyroiditis (autoimmune hypothyroidism) but there is an additional thyroid antibody at work in this disease as well, called "Thyroid Stimulating Immunoglobulin" (TSI). This additional antibody, will attach itself to the receptors that usually carry TSH to the thyroid gland and it will then mimic the stimulating action of TSH, causing the thyroid to produce and disperse more hormones of its own (T4 and T3). Graves' disease also causes swelling in the thyroid gland and so it is also known by the name "toxic diffuse goiter".

Hot nodules within the thyroid gland will mimic the action of thyroid tissue, by manufacturing and dispersing more thyroid hormones, but at an excessive rate. This is how they cause hyperthyroidism, resulting in the TSH level to drop down below the normal values range. This is sometimes called "nodular thyroid disease" and if there is also a goiter present, it is sometimes called a "nodular goiter".

TSH May Be Followed by Thyroid Blood Panels

TSH is very sensitive to even the smallest needs in either thyroid hormones. Therefore, it is so accurate in most cases of diagnosing thyroid hormone imbalances. It can detect when either hypothyroidism or hyperthyroidism is developing, sooner than any other blood test that is currently available. This is also why many doctors will first evaluate the thyroid function of their patients, using TSH alone and they will resort to testing the T4 and T3 levels, plus they will add tests to detect thyroid antibodies, when they determine that further evaluation becomes necessary. These groupings of tests are referred to as "thyroid panels" but as a far as a stand-alone test goes, TSH is by far, the best one that is currently available.

6. Nutritional Deficiencies and Hypothyroid Therapy

Patients who are diagnosed with hypothyroidism and are being treated for it with hormone replacement therapy, can sometimes have other imbalances that hinder the effectiveness of their treatment. Things such as adrenal hormones being low, ferritin/iron deficiencies, Vitamin B-12 insufficiency etc..., can cause thyroid hormone treatment, to be less-effective in patients with imbalances of these. Therefore, thorough blood and saliva testing of all levels may need to be done, to find any problems that prevent hypothyroid treatment from working as well. This is a phenomenon that happens commonly to thyroid patients who start hormone therapy however, some doctors may attribute unrelieved hypothyroid symptoms to simply being a case of a patient's body adjusting to thyroid hormone replacement medication or that unrelieved symptoms are emotional ones or psychosomatic.

Mild to moderate symptoms from adjusting to a thyroid hormone dose, should be expected but significant, unrelieved symptoms, especially those that last for weeks or longer, can mean there are other hormone imbalances or chemical imbalances needing addressed. If these are not addressed, thyroid hormone therapy may serve to intensify other hormone or nutritional imbalances. For example, thyroid hormone medication manufacturers have notations on their medication-inserts and websites, stating: "untreated adrenal cortical (cortisol) insufficiency, can worsen after beginning thyroid hormone replacement therapy".

This warning doesn't necessarily mean that patients who have a bad reaction to their thyroid medication are experiencing "true adrenal insufficiency". However, it can mean they have a degree of hypoadrenalism/adrenal fatigue (sub-clinical) or some other hormone imbalance (including sex hormones) or chemical imbalances that need correction for their hypothyroid therapy to work properly. For some patients, it can be something in the nutrient category, such as B-12 deficiency which can cause "pernicious anemia" if left untreated (thyroid patients are at higher risk for nutritional deficiencies). Unfortunately, it can require a thorough battery of blood and/or saliva lab tests to find the problem needing correction (a possible financial burden to uninsured patients).

My own doctor for example concluded a diagnosis of co-morbid CFS (Chronic Fatigue Syndrome) in my case, together with my thyroid disease, through a combination of tests, signs/symptoms and a process of elimination (extensive tests for all other possibilities). I not only had consistently low cortical (adrenal cortisol) but I was also discovered to have an unreliable TSH, in correlation with my thyroid hormone levels. My TSH remains low, even when thyroid hormones need increased, but I do not have "Central Hypothyroidism" but rather an underactive thyroid from "Hashimoto's thyroiditis". Other findings in my case included constantly swollen lymph nodes and an EBV count (Epstein-Barr Virus) that was 10 times the upper-normal cut off range on blood tests. Most thyroid patients will be found to be experiencing more easily correctable problems such as Adrenal Fatigue, low ferritin, or low B-12 etc..., when they are not seeing the expected symptom-improvement with thyroid hormone therapy alone.

Sometimes thyroid patients need their blood chemicals tested, such as electrolytes, blood gas, protein, kidney and liver enzymes, B-12 levels, adrenal hormones, sex hormones etc..., in order to zero-in on what a problem might be, if thyroid treatment is not significantly relieving certain symptoms. Mild to moderate symptoms commonly happen to well-treated hypothyroid patients but when symptoms continue, that are as severe as those found in syndromes such as CFS and Fibromyalgia, there definitely needs to be further investigation, otherwise these can seriously affect a patient's quality of life.

7. Symptoms that Merit Thyroid Blood Tests

Following are two questions generally and commonly asked by thyroid patients, with my answers following them, based on search/research I have conducted on reputable thyroid disease resource websites.

GENERAL QUESTION ONE: I suffer from severe anxiety symptoms and rapid hair loss. What type blood testing is needed and what type doctor should I seek for testing?

ANSWER: I'm sorry to hear about your very unpleasant symptoms. From the sound of it, thyroid blood tests would be a good idea because it sounds very similar to the type symptoms found in either hyperthyroid conditions or autoimmune hypothyroidism (Hashimoto's thyroiditis) which can first present with hyperthyroid symptoms.

To be honest, the type doctor doesn't matter a great deal until you first determine what area of health the symptoms represent. Any doctor who can order blood tests would be good and I would ask that he/she order a "thyroid panel" and "thyroid antibodies". Some doctors are sometimes reluctant to order thyroid antibodies until first testing thyroid hormone levels however, thyroid autoimmunity can begin causing symptoms in advance of causing abnormal thyroid hormone levels and this is why it is important that tests for them be added when symptoms match those of thyroid disease. The thyroid antibodies that can detect both autoimmune caused hypothyroid and hyperthyroidism are the "TPO, TG and TSI".

Since testing will be ordered, it is my opinion that a CBC (complete blood count) also be done and glucose level testing for diabetes. None of the tests are very expensive and would help to rule out other possibilities and help to zero in on the problem.

GENERAL QUESTION TWO: After treatment for hypothyroidism for 20 years, I've lately experienced a return of hypothyroid symptoms and requiring frequent dose changes over the past several months, why is this happening?

ANSWER: My suspicion is that with your doctor watching your blood lab levels, he can see that you're entering a phase of needing dose increases. He should be able to get you leveled out again over time. I've heard of this before, when patients seem to reach a point that their own thyroids finally fizzle out or at least reach a more significant point of damage and non-functioning with hypothyroidism.

When we take thyroid hormone medication, it is to aid our own thyroid glands in supplying needed hormones but over time, it does actually replace the thyroid gland completely, once it reaches its expected death from years of auto-antibodies attacking it. As you are treated, you might ask for copies of your blood retest lab reports and discuss anything with your doctor you see in them that you feel might improve your results (e.g. a change in dose or in the type/brand of medication).

8. Taking Thyroid Medication Before a Blood Draw

TSH is the most common test used to monitor hypothyroid patients who are treated with thyroid hormone replacement therapy (Thyroid Stimulating Hormone). As thyroid hormone is increased (higher doses), the TSH level drops and rises when thyroid hormone is decreased (lower doses). An above-normal -- abnormally high TSH indicates hypothyroidism, when a patient is first diagnosed.

The question of whether a hypothyroid patient should take their thyroid hormone medication-dose before each blood draw, that is done to monitor their replacement therapy is a common one. Patients wonder if taking the hormone dose will affect lab results, when taken only an hour or two before the blood is drawn for a retest of their treatment hormone levels. In most cases, I feel any slight change this would cause in blood lab results would not be significant enough, to result in a doctor changing a patient's treatment (e.g. increasing or decreasing their dose).

When dose adjustments are need, these can be done even at small increments. The thyroid hormone replacement drug "Synthroid" (synthetic T4 only brand) for example, has dose levels that can be adjusted at 12mcg increments or higher and "Armour Thyroid" (natural combo of T4 and T3) can be adjusted at 15mg increments or higher.

The timing of a patient's dose in correlation with blood draws for retesting their treatment hormone levels, is not usually significant unless they are the type patient, whose dose must be kept within a very narrow margin-level. There are, however, statements made by the manufacturer of Armour Thyroid, recommending that patients on the day of retesting, should not take their hormone dose before blood draw, but that they should wait to take it after blood has been drawn.

Here is a short quote:

"If you are on a thyroid supplement medication and need to take a blood test, on the day of your blood test, you should wait to take your medication until after your blood has been drawn to avoid any test interference."

(From the "Diagnosis" page of the Armour Thyroid website, under the heading "Blood Tests").

Whether you decide to take your thyroid hormone dose before or after your blood is drawn for retests, this is a decision that should be made between you and your doctor. The main thing is to be consistent in whatever method you use, and this will insure consistency in each of your blood retest lab results.

9. Thyroid Autoimmunity and Temporary Thyroiditis

Having "thyroiditis", simply means your thyroid gland has become inflamed. Some of the reasons for thyroiditis, include viral illnesses, recovering from child birthing and permanent autoimmunity.

There are several terms available, to describe a variety of causes and manifestations of an inflamed thyroid gland or what is medically referred to as "thyroiditis". There are temporary types of thyroiditis including one called "Viral thyroiditis" -- also refer to as "DeQuervain's thyroiditis" (usually caused by upper respiratory illnesses) and if it is painful to the thyroid gland, it is referred to as "Sub-Acute thyroiditis". If it is not painful, they call it "Silent Thyroiditis" -- this is often the type experienced by women, following pregnancy or what is also referred to as "postpartum thyroiditis".

Woman Experience Thyroiditis Far More Often Than Do Men

As I begin the paragraph for this subheading, I will mention that I am one of the relatively rare cases of a man with hypothyroidism from autoimmune thyroiditis. Some medical statistics have shown that thyroid diseases and disorders, are from 8 to 10 times more common in women than in men. One reason for the large difference in the frequency of occurrence of thyroiditis in women, is pregnancy. Medical statistics have shown that up to 25% of women will develop some degree of thyroiditis, within one year following giving birth, which is referred to as "postpartum thyroiditis". In most cases, the thyroiditis will first cause symptoms of hyperthyroidism (overactive gland- sped up metabolism) and before ending within a few weeks, it will transition over to hypothyroidism (underactive gland – slowed down metabolism). In most cases, both conditions usually resolve on their own, however, up to 20% of women who develop postpartum thyroiditis, will end up with permanent autoimmune hypothyroidism, that requires lifelong treatment.

Thyroid Autoimmunity May Surface Following Viral Thyroiditis

While many people who experience one of these temporary types of viral thyroiditis, have no problems afterward, once it resolves within a few weeks, others who experience them go on to develop autoimmune thyroiditis, also referred to as "Hashimoto's disease". This type is not temporary but is rather permanent and usually requires lifelong treatment with thyroid hormone replacement medication, due to the progressive hypothyroidism it causes. Another medical term for the permanent type, is "Chronic Lymphocytic Thyroiditis". It is also the most common cause of a low-functioning thyroid gland, in the U.S. and in most other industrialized countries.

It's possible that those who experience a case of viral thyroiditis, already have the beginnings or "early onset" of Hashimoto's developing in their bodies when the viral illness was contracted (dormant but on the verge of manifesting) and this hastens the onset of permanent thyroid autoimmunity. A doctor can diagnose Hashimoto's, through blood testing of "thyroid antibodies" levels. These are the killer cells from the immune system, that are sent to destroy the thyroid gland, once becoming misdirected -- mistakenly recognizing the thyroid gland as a threat to the body. They normally attack germs and allergens, in order to eradicate them from the body, so that any illness we experience from them is limited in duration and strength.

A Theory for Why Thyroid Autoimmunity Occurs

They refer to immune cell attacks on normal bodily organs, as "autoimmune disease", when the body turns on itself and attacks part of its own natural tissues. One theory for the cause of autoimmunity, is that the immune system recognizes a part of the body as an intruder because of a virus that has settled into its tissues. The immune system is attempting to fully eradicate the virus from the body. For it to do this, it mistakenly believes it has to attack the tissues that contain or that are holding the virus. Over time the immune system is successful in damaging and ultimately destroying these tissues, which can include the thyroid gland, resulting in hypothyroidism -- a low functioning gland.

The main antibodies that cause autoimmune hypothyroidism (Hashimoto's), are the "anti-thyroid peroxidase" (anti-TPO) and the "anti-thyroglobulin" (anti-TG). If a person tests positive for either or both antibodies (also called "auto-antibodies"), via blood testing, this would confirm Hashimoto's Disease/thyroiditis as a cause of hypothyroidism. There is also a thyroid tissue biopsy that can be performed, called an FNA (Fine Needle Aspiration) and this is also a definitive test for diagnosing Hashimoto's.

Ordering Thyroid Antibody and Hormone Panels

Doctors may test patients who develop thyroiditis, for low thyroid hormone levels, to see if hypothyroidism has already begun. A "thyroid Panel", that includes the "TSH" level and the "Free T-4" and possibly also the "Free T-3", can determine how far-along a case of thyroiditis may be in causing hypothyroidism. Some patients have the permanent type of disease but their thyroid hormones and TSH level (Thyroid Stimulating Hormone) are within normal range. They may still experience a degree of symptoms however, despite hypothyroidism not being evident on blood labs. This is a fact that has been confirmed in several medical research studies. Some doctors will start these patients on a small dose of thyroid hormone replacement medication if thyroid autoimmunity is present and causing early hypothyroid symptoms.

Doctors should order the anti-TPO and anti-TG antibodies blood tests, along with a thyroid hormone panel when evaluating a patient suspected of having hypothyroid disease. If a doctor is not willing to order these highly diagnostic tests, a patient should find one who is willing to order them, so that early-onset thyroid disease is not overlooked. This particular statement also comes from my own personal experience, when proper blood tests were not ordered initially in my case, at a time when I was suffering from depression, anxiety, joint aches, dry skin and severe fatigue (symptoms highly indicative of hypothyroidism). Once these tests were ordered, my thyroid disease was clearly revealed.

Patients Know When Their Bodies Feel Abnormal

My thyroid disease was only properly diagnosed, once I demanded the proper blood tests, designed to detect thyroid antibodies and abnormal thyroid hormone levels. My doctor at the time, was attempting to convince me that my symptoms were emotional or psychosomatic. However, I knew that I had a physical, medical problem occurring, in need of being diagnosed. In my case, both my thyroid panel and the associated antibodies tests were abnormal and thyroid hormone replacement therapy was highly effective in relieving my initial symptoms, once being administered to me by a specialized thyroid doctor.

When symptoms of thyroid inflammation are occurring, which can include swelling in the thyroid gland area (the front of the neck, just below the Adams Apple) or pain that is coming from that same area, or if there is difficulty with swallowing, it is important that consultation with a qualified medical doctor, is sought as soon as possible.

10. Thyroid Disease a Risk for Related Conditions

Some years ago on the Thyroid Health forum, a member asked a question in regard to "co-morbid conditions" that can develop along with thyroid disease, which I explained was another term for "related conditions" (other health disorders or diseases that are strongly associated with thyroid diseases). I took the opportunity in my reply on that thread, to list what I believe are important blood tests for thyroid patients to have done, when they are experiencing symptoms that might indicate a co-morbid condition has developed or is developing.

Certainly, thyroid patients should also proactively make sure they are under the care of a doctor who is optimizing their thyroid disease treatment, so that inadequate - lack of proper treatment can first be ruled out as a cause of their unresolved symptoms. Following below, is the edited reply I posted on the forum thread about conditions that can be co-morbid/related to thyroid diseases and the blood tests that can detect them. ---

Co-morbid conditions are also called "related Conditions" and you can read lots of articles I have under several headings on the Thyroid Health website (left column of Homepage). These headings include: "Physical Conditions", "Anxiety-Depression", "Metabolic Conditions" and "Fatigued Adrenals".

In most of the articles, I have suggestions for being properly tested for these related conditions. I will say in general, that I feel thyroid patients should be thoroughly worked up on blood labs, such as getting a CBC (complete blood count) which checks for anemia and other blood abnormalities, an A1C (glucose average for 2 to 3 months), which checks for diabetes, a Lipid Panel (includes cholesterol and triglycerides levels) and a Metabolic Panel (kidney, liver, and electrolytes).

I also believe adrenal hormone and sex hormone testing should be done as well, to check for any imbalances that might be present in those, such as adrenal fatigue, menopause, hyperandrogenism (abnormally high male hormones in females) and PCOS (Polycystic Ovarian Syndrome).

If a patient has inflammatory symptoms like joint/muscle pain, blood tests that check for systemic inflammation (significant-widespread) and systemic autoimmunity should be ordered, such as ANA, ESR, CRP and Rheumatoid Factor. These can help detect autoimmune arthritis, connective tissue diseases, Lupus and other autoimmune diseases. If a CBC reveals anemia, the vitamin B-12 level should then be tested, to distinguish between iron and vitamin deficiency as the cause. I feel it is a good idea to get B-12 tested regardless because low B-12 is the cause of pernicious anemia (also an autoimmune disease) and it can drop to very low levels, before it is revealed in a CBC as anemia. Meanwhile, unresolved fatigue would likely be a prominent symptom.

These are just some suggestions to consider but the most important thing is that patients tell their doctors about any unresolved symptoms they're having and to also search/research online, about conditions that might be responsible (one should always use reputable, reliable medical websites). This helps patients discuss possible testing that might be needed, with their doctors. Despite what some observers of patient proactive-ness might believe to the contrary, many doctors do like this type of cooperative-input by their patients. In many cases, this can help them to zero-in on the cause of unresolved symptoms that a well-treated thyroid patient is still experiencing.

11. Treating Thyroid Hormone Conversion Failure

Patients, who are treated for hypothyroidism, sometimes are found to have "impaired T-4 to T-3 conversion". These are patients who for some reason, do not have the ability within their body to adequately convert enough T-4 into the more-needed T-3 hormone. Doctors do not always identify the problem that results in impaired conversion, but it may at times be due to an inability of the liver to aid in the conversion process (usually due to liver disease).

There may also be co-morbid (co-existing) illness or disease of other kinds in the body that hinder the conversion process of T-4 to T-3. Regardless of the cause that may or may not be found, these patients will need to have the low T-3 hormone replaced with thyroid hormone replacement therapy that includes both T-4 and T-3, rather than with a T-4 only thyroid hormone medication.

Most patients with hypothyroidism are prescribed a T-4 only brand of thyroid hormone medication and the needed T-3 hormone is converted from it, within the body successfully. In patients with the less common "impaired conversion" however, a T-4 only hormone medication will not supply them with adequate T-3 that is also needed in the body.

Unfortunately, some doctors do not believe impaired conversion of T-4 to T-3 happens, except in extremely rare cases. This will result in less blood testing of treated hypothyroid patients, of their T-4 and T-3 levels because it will be deemed unnecessary. Doctors will often only monitor hypothyroid patients on T-4 only hormone treatments, using a TSH test only.

The TSH or "Thyroid Stimulating Hormone" is not a thyroid hormone but is a pituitary hormone as that reflects how much thyroid hormone is available in the body, via the blood stream. The problem however, with not testing both T-4 and T-3 levels in patients treated with a T-4 only medications, at least for the first one or two follow up retests, is that adequate T-4 in the blood will give often give a normal TSH reading even when the T-3 hormone is low.

In my opinion as a layperson and treated hypothyroid patient who has extensively researched this subject and corresponded with many treated hypothyroid patients, blood retests need to include the "Free T-4" and "Free T-3" levels (the "free levels" are the tests of unbound, available hormone). This would be in addition to TSH, for at least the first two blood retests in follow up on T-4 only thyroid hormone replacement therapy.

If these first follow up tests indicate that hormone replacement is resulting in adequate amounts of both T-4 and T-3 (proper conversion), Then TSH only testing would be enough for follow up retests, afterward.

12. TSH Blood Test Considerations

There has been ongoing debate in regard to TSH blood testing, both in regard to diagnosing and treating hypothyroidism (the best normal values for each). There are still top qualified Endocrinologists and MDs who believe anything below a "2.0" TSH, is a risky treatment-level (a level they believe could lead to thyrotoxicity -- dose induced hyperthyroidism) while others believe that 1.0 should be the target-goal for TSH suppression via a thyroid hormone replacement dose to treat hypothyroidism. TSH elevates with hypothyroidism and suppresses when thyroid hormones are increased (the purpose of hypothyroid, hormone drug therapy).

The unfortunate thing is that these type issues, leave patients with the need to try different trials of dosing until they find a level that brings them the most symptom relief. It is certainly important to have a doctor behind thyroid medication trials if possible (this may depend on what country you live in -- doctor availability). I'm thankful my doctor is completely behind me in my hypothyroid treatment and her main concern is the same as mine, which is to make sure I stay within best normal values on my T4 and T3 levels, regardless of any trial of T4 or T3 medication I might take (e.g. higher dose trials, when my blood retests show that I need a dose increase). My TSH is not accurate in reflecting my thyroid hormone levels, which is unusual. This was determined early-on in my hormone therapy, so thankfully in my case I'm not tied down to TSH testing. In most patients TSH does reflect their thyroid hormone levels accurately.

These type scenarios and others are what make it difficult for even the most reputable medical research groups to pin areas of thyroid disease treatments down to an exact science (unfortunate but true) and this is largely due to "patient-individuality". There are too many variables that cause patients to have different results from same hypothyroid treatment trials. The TSH issue for example, can include the questions of whether a patient has a goitrous or non-goitrous condition, cold nodules, hot nodules and co-morbid disease-processes that may change the reliability of TSH among different patients. I've stated many times in the past, that medical treatment developments influenced by medical research groups, is a job I would not want to have! It has mountains of difficulty involved with it, but we are certainly thankful for the advances they have already brought us!

Because of the different types of thyroid hormone brands that might be used and because of the possibility that TSH may not be accurate in all treated hypothyroid patients, it is important that follow-up, blood retesting of treatment hormone levels, includes T4, T3 and TSH -- especially in newly treated patients.

13. My Review For: The Thyroid Diet Revolution

This is my book review for Mary Shomon's book on increasing metabolism, for improved weight loss/control. This New York Times best seller is a great resource for thyroid patients seeking diet advice.

In "The Thyroid Diet Revolution: Manage Your Master Gland of Metabolism for Lasting Weight Loss" -- a book by Thyroid Patient Advocate - Mary Shomon, one of the most concerning problem-areas for thyroid patients is addressed. The problem so amply covered by the author, "is weight gain and difficulty losing weight", due to a hypothyroid metabolism. I was graciously provided a free review copy of this New York Times bestseller, by the author - Mrs. Mary J. Shomon.

Hypothyroid Metabolism

Having a slowed metabolic rate in the body, is a common complaint heard from treated thyroid patients who find that it requires a great deal more effort for them to control their weight, than before they experienced the onset of thyroid disease. As a male hypothyroid patient, I too can attest to an ongoing struggle with weight loss/control but I also see the added importance in addressing this problem with the fact that thyroid patients are at higher risk for other metabolic related diseases, including diabetes.

These are the reasons this book is such an important resource for thyroid patients to take advantage of.

Looking at Mary's book, she begins by covering information on the symptoms, diagnosis and treatments for thyroid conditions because a weight problem can arise in people who are unaware that they have thyroid conditions. This part of the book looks at risk factors for thyroid disease, missed cases of thyroid dysfunction due to improper testing to detect it and people who have borderline thyroid conditions that doctors may not be willing to treat. All thyroid conditions are discussed in this section of the book, including hypothyroidism (under-active thyroid), hyperthyroidism (some hyperthyroid treatments result in hypothyroidism), goiter, nodules and thyroid cancer and how these are also treated.

She also includes information on challenges that may arise in getting properly diagnosed due to doctors who may not order all the necessary tests. She points out that in addition to TSH, tests for thyroid antibodies (for thyroid autoimmunity) and testing of Reverse T3 and TRH (Thyrotropin Releasing Hormone) to monitor conversion of T4 into T3 in the body may also be needed. Mary discusses treatment for hypothyroidism and looks at the different types of thyroid hormone replacement therapies that are available and the importance of optimized treatment for best results. Good nutrition and natural supplements are addressed, including vitamins, minerals and other natural helps that can be incorporated into treatment for hypothyroidism. It was great to see information included on things you should avoid in your diet, including "goitrogen foods" (listed in the book) which can contribute to goiter and reduced thyroid hormone levels.

Continuing in the book, Mary gives wonderful, easy-to-understand but detailed explanation describing the metabolic process of food being converted into energy for the body (metabolism and gluconeogenesis). She includes information on the role of insulin, glucagon, leptin, ghrelin, cortisol and adrenaline (metabolic hormones) in this process and how imbalances developing in these delicately balanced hormones, can lead to problems with weight gain and health disorders, including metabolic syndrome and diabetes.

She goes on to describe what it means to be "metabolically efficient", meaning you strike a proper balance between the proper foods you eat, proper aerobic exercise, proper nutrition and hydration and taking into account menopause, which can highly effect hormonal balance in affected women. Inflammatory response in the body is also discussed and how it can point to hormonal imbalance and affect weight control in the body (an aspect I found highly interesting).

Proper Dieting Plans

Mary helps readers to look at options for developing the best possible diet plan for their individual needs. These sections contain informative graphs breaking down the details of each diet plan and includes a check list that helps you determine the best diet for you as an individual. A Body Mass Index is also included to help you determine your best weight level in setting a realistic goal to achieve your desired weight. The nice thing about these sections is that you can try different options if one doesn't work the desired results for you.

She also suggests lots of recipes with a breakdown chart for each, showing the amounts of calories, fats, carbohydrates, fiber, sugar and protein they contain. She also points out foods high in protein, those that are low-glycemic (low sugar, starch and fat) and provides a chart that distinguishes between beneficial and non-beneficial fats. Also found are suggestions on how to determine the size portions you eat of the foods you choose, the importance of including proper amounts of fiber, water and positive hope/attitude. She includes chapters on more specialized diets and procedures that patients may consider when weight loss is especially difficult, including prescription weight loss drugs when needed. She also helps us identify those things we need to avoid in our diets, including alcohol, caffeine, refined sugars and some artificial sweeteners.

I am personally implementing the suggestions in Mary's book, into my own dieting practices. As previously-mentioned, my weight control has become far more difficult for me, since my hypothyroidism diagnoses in 2003, plus I am now in my 50s and this has naturally affected my metabolism as well, Additionally, I'm taking a prescription drug for peripheral neuropathy (idiopathic – non-diabetic), that has "weight gain" as a listed side effect for it. With these issues occurring in my life, I must give special attention to my weight gain issue otherwise I make myself vulnerable to developing additional health condition, such as diabetes, heart disease and types of cancer that obese individuals are at higher risk for developing.

Overcoming Weight Gain Culprits

Mary further addresses weight loss issues (hindrances), giving further attention to blood sugar balance, the effects of allergies (including food intolerances) and toxins on metabolism. I was especially interested in the included information on the adrenal hormone imbalance subject, where she discusses "Adrenal Fatigue" which occurs commonly in thyroid patients. A common fungus overgrowth problem (yeast infection) is also discussed which is caused by the candida fungus, referred to as "Candidiasis" and can be a result of too much refined sugar in the diet. Mary discusses treatments for this yeast overgrowth that can hinder weight loss, including diet changes and natural supplements that can help including probiotics and anti-fungal drugs required in more severe cases.

Another common health disorder negatively affecting digestion and the body's ability to absorb nutrients is addressed, called "Celiac Disease" -- a chronic disorder caused by an allergy to gluten (wheat, barley, rye and possibly oat products). Mary points out that even without having this disease, people can be gluten intolerant with similar negative results and that if it is suspected, tests to diagnose the problem may be needed so that a gluten-free diet can be started to help in recovery and prevention of the disease-effects. She also points out that parasites (parasitic infections) can have negative effects on metabolism and weight control, as can an imbalance between zinc and copper levels in the body. Tests that can determine a patient's status in these areas are discussed as are treatments and diet-change options to resolve the problems when found.

Mary includes information on prescription drugs that can contribute to weight gain and lists several natural supplements that can help with weight loss. Also included is a look at mind-body and spiritual aspects that can contribute to overall balance of health. She also goes into the subject of stress, anxiety and depression (these can also affect metabolism) and gives an overview in regard to prescription drugs that can be administered for problems in this area, when they are resistant to natural supplements, diet and exercise. Cognitive Behavioral Therapy (CBT) is included as a subject as well as self-help relaxation techniques, deep breathing, Emotional Freedom Techniques (EFT) and other stress reducers. She also gives a great run down in regard to exercise, things that can hinder your ability to get proper exercise and how to overcome those and benefit the best possible from a proper exercise regimen.

A Highly Recommended Book

It's hard to know where to stop in this review because there is so much great information in this book and I've barely scratched the surface. I'll simply end in saying it is a great overall resource to help thyroid patients develop an effective weight loss plan and diet for improved health and quality-of-life. With so many suggestions and options included, you're sure to find the right plan for weight loss and weight control in this remarkable book and I highly recommend it.

I offer my sincere thanks to Mrs. Shomon, for providing me the free book copy and for placing faith in me, to provide an adequate published review for it. The book is available at all major bookseller websites and stores.

SECTION THREE

Essential Thyroid Disorder Basic Information

TABLE OF CONTENTS:

1. Actions of Thyroid Hormones

Thyroid hormone metabolism involves iodine, TSH, T4, T3, Reverse T3 and the thyroid gland. When this metabolic process takes place properly, correct levels of energy are supplied to cells of the body.

Thyroid hormone metabolism in the body, is a process in which the thyroid gland absorbs iodine from foods consumed and then converts that element into hormones that reach every cell in the body, to provide them energy.

Common Hypothyroid and Hyperthyroid Disorders

If too much thyroid hormone is being manufactured and dispersed into the body, "hyperthyroidism" will be the result -- a term meaning one has an overactive thyroid gland. If an insufficient amount of thyroid hormone is being produced and sent-out to the cells of the body, "hypothyroidism" will occur -- meaning one has an underactive thyroid gland. Most cases of thyroid hormone disorders (imbalances), have common causes, such as thyroid autoimmunity (immune cells attacking the thyroid gland), old age, pregnancy, toxic chemical exposure and iodine deficiency.

Within the first four subheadings following below, the proper steps that occur during normal thyroid hormone metabolism, will be described. In the final, 5th subheading, an uncommon hypothyroid condition from an overabundance of "Reverse T3 conversion", will be briefly discussed.

Iodine is Converted into Thyroid Hormones

The thyroid is mostly comprised of an element called "iodine". The iodine is first absorbed from the diet by the thyroid gland and then converted into energy for the body, through cells called hormones -- each containing a certain number of iodine molecules within them. These thyroid hormones are sent from the thyroid gland, throughout the body, to regulate the metabolism -- the rate at which the body functions when burning energies (food water and oxygen). The two major thyroid hormones are the "T-4" and the "T-3" and blood levels of these are tested to detect abnormally low or abnormally high levels, caused by thyroid hormone imbalances-disorders.

TSH Regulates Thyroid Hormone Production

Another major hormone is also blood-tested to evaluate thyroid function, called "TSH" (Thyroid Stimulating Hormone). This one comes from the pituitary gland and so it is not actually a thyroid hormone. This master gland in the brain monitors and regulates the thyroid, which means the blood TSH level, gives an accurate reflective measure of how well the thyroid is functioning, in producing its own hormones. TSH goes the opposite direction and becomes low when the thyroid is overactive (when thyroid hormones are abnormally high) and it becomes high when it is under-active (when thyroid hormones are abnormally low).

Conversion of T4 into T3

The T-4 hormone contains four iodine molecules and another name for it is "thyroxine". It is more abundant and found in larger supply in the body than is the T-3 hormone, also called "triiodothyronine", which only contains three iodine molecules. Even though T-4 contains one more iodine molecule, T-3 is at least five times more powerful than T-4. The T-4 hormone is the less metabolically active of the two and is stored in the body and converted into the more active T-3 hormone, as it is needed in the body for metabolism. This conversion process is accomplished via enzymes and proteins found in the body which attach to the T-4 hormone cells, turning them into T-3 hormone, as the body needs it to burn higher levels of energy. This conversion process takes place within the liver and partially within the kidneys as well.

"Reverse T3" Prevents T3 and T4 Toxicity (Hyperthyroidism)

When there is excess T-4 in the body, it is not converted into T-3 but instead it will be converted into a substance called "Reverse T-3". This is how the body rids itself of extra T-4 in the body that is in excess to the amount needed to be stored and converted into T-3. Reverse T-3 is a term meaning the excess T-4 hormone has been rendered inactive, so that too much of it is not converted into T-3 which would cause an overactive metabolism or a type of hyperthyroidism (also referred to as "thyrotoxicity").

Low T3 Syndromes

Certain types of illnesses and severe, chronic stress, can cause the body to convert too much of the T-4 hormone into Reverse T-3, which will cause a person to experience a type of "hypothyroidism" (under-active thyroid), due to low T-3 in the body. This type of hypothyroidism that is secondary to an illness or stress in the body is also referred to as "Euthyroid Sick

Syndrome" or sometimes it is referred to as "Wilson's Temperature Syndrome". It is usually a temporary form of hypothyroidism that can be corrected with short term T-3 hormone replacement therapy. This type of hypothyroidism is rare compared to the types that are caused by a diseased thyroid gland or what is also known as "primary hypothyroidism". It is also rare compared to the type of underactive thyroid caused by disease or dysfunction of the glands that help regulate thyroid function (the pituitary and hypothalamus), which is referred to as "Secondary Hypothyroidism" or "Central Hypothyroidism".

Thyroid hormone metabolism is an amazing process, involving a number of different elements, proteins and enzymes, working together to manufacture these amazing cells called "thyroid hormones", that supply us with the needed energy to perform our daily activities, throughout our lives.

2. Basic Facts about Goiters

When a thyroid patient has a goiter, this simply means they have swelling of the thyroid gland, which is located at the front of the neck in the area just below the Adam's apple. Goiters are recognized as different types and for affecting part of the thyroid, such as one of the two lobes or the middle part of the gland called the isthmus or for affecting the entire gland. They are also considered different types depending upon the causes of them. A major cause of goiters are autoimmune thyroid diseases.

If a goiter is caused by iodine deficiency, it is referred to as a "colloid nodular" or "endemic' goiter. This type is rare in the U.S. and many other industrialized countries that use iodized table salt, which usually provides those that consume it, enough iodine to avoid iodine deficiency hypothyroidism and the resulting endemic goiters.

If a person's thyroid gland has swelling plus several small tumors called "nodules" within it, they refer to this type as a "multi-nodular goiter". Nodules within a gland that has goiter can be the type that causes the gland to produce excess thyroid hormone, in which case they will add the term "toxic" to the term, calling it a "toxic multi-nodular goiter". People with Hashimoto's thyroiditis commonly have mild multi-nodular goiters that are non-toxic. When a person is termed as having a "diffuse goiter", this means there is general swelling throughout the gland that is not caused by nodules. This type of goiter can also cause toxicity or over-activity of the thyroid gland (hyperthyroidism), in which case it is referred to as a "toxic diffuse goiter". These types are found commonly in patients with Grave's Disease.

Temporary types of thyroiditis, such as those that occur with viral infections and in pregnant women can also cause goiter (asymmetrical enlargement) but these types will usually resolve within a few weeks, along with the thyroiditis. These type goiters can flare short-term with these types of thyroiditis and cause severe pain in the thyroid gland, which is referred to as "sub-acute thyroiditis", while other types do not cause a painful thyroid which is referred to as "silent thyroiditis".

A goiter can be mild, so that it is barely visible by looking at the affected person's neck or sometimes not visible at all with the naked eye. The same is true of detecting a goiter by human feel or what they refer to as "palpation". Some cannot be felt or seen but may still have enough swelling, present within them to cause mild discomfort and a mild feeling of inflammation in the neck. When goiters become severe, they can become large enough to obstruct swallowing and breathing and, in these cases, thyroid removal (total-thyroidectomy) might be an option a treating doctor would consider. When goiters are less severe, treating any thyroid hormone imbalance that is present in the patient can help to shrink them and prevent further growth.

Patients, who have goiters or are suspected of having them, may be referred for a "thyroid ultrasound" (sound-wave imaging/sonogram) or a "thyroid uptake scan" (radiology/radioactive iodine) and possibly even an MRI (Magnetic Resonance Imaging). These are diagnostic tests that give detailed images of the thyroid gland, to determine the size of goiters and whether they contain nodules within them that are not detectable by palpation.

If you feel tightness or swelling in your throat in the area of the thyroid gland or you can actually see visible swelling, report to your doctor for a checkup and evaluation of your symptoms, making sure to list any other symptoms you are having, in detail. Most goiters can be treated, so that any symptoms they are causing are improved or significantly relieved.

3. Basics about Thyroid Disease Symptoms

Shown below, are two lists of symptoms. One is a general list of symptoms that may indicate hypothyroidism -- an under-functioning thyroid gland. The second list are the general symptoms that may indicate hyperthyroidism -- an over-active thyroid gland. Eighty percent of thyroid hormone imbalances that are diagnosed, are in the hypothyroid category (the other 20% are hyperthyroid). Most thyroid hormone disorders are caused by autoimmune disease of the thyroid gland.

What are the main symptoms of "hypothyroidism"?

1. Tiredness, fatigue, lack of energy and stamina

2. Depressed mood, at times alternating with anxiety

3. Dry skin that flakes and dry brittle hair that tends to fall out

4. Constipation from slowed digestion

5. Slowed heart rate, hypotension and at times hypertension

6. Moderate weight gain from slowed metabolism

7. Goiter or nodules (small tumors) of the thyroid gland

(These symptoms can increase in severity without treatment to restore bodily metabolism -- thyroid hormone replacement therapy.)

What are the main symptoms of "hyperthyroidism" (generally opposite from Hypothyroidism symptoms)?

1. Excessive energy, feeling keyed-up and nervous (resulting in fatigue)

2. Anxious mood, at times alternating with depression

3. Oily skin and hair, excessive sweating

4. Diarrhea

5. Weight loss from increased metabolism

6. Rapid heart rate and hypertension

7. Eyes that bulge or that seem exaggeratedly wide-open

8. Goiter or nodules of the thyroid gland

(These symptoms can also become severe if left untreated -- e.g. heart and blood pressure effects. Treatments include medications to slow thyroid hormone production and hyper-metabolism or thyroid removal.)

People who experience a number of these symptoms or even one of them that is concerning for possible thyroid disease, need to see their doctor for a checkup and evaluation. Thyroid hormone imbalances are usually first detected by blood testing and a patient presenting with symptoms of either hypothyroidism or hyperthyroidism, may be referred for a blood draw to test their thyroid function (usually via a "thyroid panel" or a "TSH test" alone).

4. Basics about Thyroid Nodules

Thyroid nodules are small tumor-like growths on the thyroid gland. According to statistics, as much as 10 percent of the general population has thyroid nodules but they occur far more often in thyroid diseases. People with autoimmune thyroid diseases have abnormal thyroid tissue and over time can develop many nodules or what is referred to as "multi-nodules". Thyroid nodules can be detected by feel or "palpation" but some may be in an area of the gland that are only detectable by diagnostic imaging tests such as "thyroid ultrasound" (sound wave imaging), "Radio Active Iodine Uptake Scans" (radiological imaging) and "MRI" (Magnetic Resonance Imaging).

Thyroid nodules that are solitary or found to be one, have a slightly higher risk of containing cancer cells (malignancy) than do multi-nodules and larger nodules are also considered more suspicious. When a solitary nodule is located, the treating doctor may wish to have a tissue biopsy performed. The procedure that is usually performed to obtain a thyroid nodule tissue sample is called a "Fine Needle Aspiration" (FNA) and is a simple out-patient procedure.

The tissue sample is then lab-analyzed to detect any abnormal cells indicating the presence of either "papillary" or "follicular" cancer, which are the two major types that can potentially invade the thyroid gland. Fortunately, should cancer cells be detected, thyroid cancers have a very high treatment success rate. Treatment of benign thyroid nodules involves removal of the thyroid gland (total thyroidectomy) and administering full thyroid hormone replacement therapy for that patient as a lifelong treatment afterward.

When thyroid nodules are being investigated, they may be placed into several categories. We have already looked at solitary and multi-nodules but other terms used in describing them include "hot nodules", meaning the nodule is actively absorbing iodine from the thyroid gland and is releasing thyroid hormone, causing a hormone imbalance in the patient (hyperthyroidism). Smaller hot nodules may not cause hyperthyroidism while larger ones usually do, and many times are also biopsied due to their larger size. If the nodule is not causing thyroid hormone release, it is referred to as a "cold nodule" and both hot and cold nodules have a distinct appearance on diagnostic imaging tests.

Some thyroid nodules are more solid than others which are referred to as "solid nodules" and these are also considered more suspicious of possibly containing cancer cells and may also be biopsied as a precaution, depending upon their size. Many non-solid nodules are "cystic nodules" because they will contain fluid in the center of them and these types, are almost never considered a risk for containing cancer cells.

While this gives us a basic understanding of most types of thyroid nodules and how they more-commonly manifest, there are always the possibilities of crossover features. In other words, some are not as easily distinguishable as being of a specific type and may have features of several types (complex nodule). If you find that you have a growth/tumor or several growths on your thyroid gland, it is important that you see your doctor for an evaluation of them. She will likely thoroughly palpate your thyroid gland (feel by fingertips) and if she determines that the nodules need further evaluation, may also send you for a thyroid ultrasound or uptake scan. These will help determine whether there is a need to have any nodules biopsied, as a precaution against developing thyroid cancer.

5. Iodine a Factor in Hypothyroidism?

Sometime ago I was corresponding with a friend, who related to me that he was experiencing symptoms that were suspicious of being thyroid hormone related. His father had been diagnosed with thyroid disease years earlier, plus his Doctor, who referred him to an Endocrinologist, also felt that his symptoms needed further evaluation for possible thyroid involvement. He posed some questions to me regarding his iodine intake and regarding the fact that his blood lab test levels of iodine came back slightly elevated. He also asked if his symptoms of swelling in different tissue-areas of his body and exercise intolerance were possibly related to undiagnosed thyroid dysfunction.

Below was my general response to my friend:

I don't often hear of people getting their blood iodine levels checked because iodine doesn't necessarily tell you anything about your thyroid function. Iodine can elevate in the body due to what is in your diet (high iodine foods like kelp and other types of edible seaweeds) or because of supplements you take that contain high iodine content. The real tests of thyroid function are the actual thyroid hormone levels, called "T-4 and T-3" and the one called "TSH" which is a pituitary hormone but is sensitive in reflecting thyroid function, when blood levels are tested.

Regarding high iodine content foods or supplements containing iodine, I would suggest not consuming these until after you are evaluated for thyroid function. Iodine can work adversely in people with "autoimmune thyroid disease", which is the most common cause of low thyroid hormone imbalance, in most industrialized countries. Let me add however, that iodine is the treatment for hypothyroidism caused by iodine deficiency, but this type is almost non-existent in industrialized countries. Use of iodized salt alone (table salt) usually contains as much iodine as average, healthy people need for thyroid function.

Your symptoms of feeling flu-like and swelling (edema) after hard physical activity could possibly be thyroid related. This is especially true if you have a parent or sibling who has thyroid disease because it does run in families. You are possibly experiencing symptoms from the onset of "autoimmune thyroid disease". This type can potentially cause symptoms even before thyroid hormone levels become abnormal. It is diagnosed via "thyroid antibodies" blood tests. These are the "anti-TPO", "anti-TG" and sometimes the "TSI" antibody levels. If any of these come back positive, this will mean that you have thyroid autoimmunity, meaning your own immune system is attacking your thyroid gland.

I'm glad to hear that you are going to an Endocrinologist because most are better specialized in diagnosing and treating thyroid disorders. The thyroid gland is part of the Endocrine System, meaning it is one of the glands that supplies our bodies with needed hormones. An Endo or a Thyroid Specialist are two doctors that I suggest to people needing thyroid evaluation or even an MD who is highly experienced in treating thyroid disorders and diseases.

6. Men Get Thyroid Disease Too!

Below is information I shared with a friend of mine -- a man who described to me symptoms he was experiencing from hypothyroidism. He was experiencing the typical hypothyroid symptoms but the two of most concern to him were his emotional ones and his diminished libido (sex drive). Following below are some of the things I shared in response to him.

"The titration (dose adjustments) of your thyroid medication can take several changes over several months, before they get you to a good euthyroid state (normal hormone levels). It's hard to be "patient" with the process but we have no choice. Also, while you might be a patient that sees very good resolution of symptoms with thyroid hormone therapy, many of us have somewhat satisfactory relief but never reach 100% of what we were before experiencing hypothyroid disease. I've had many improvements myself, but I still experience flares of fatigue, brain fog etc... These are improved in many ways and less frequent, since being treated.

The libido problem should also improve for you over time. I almost completely lost interest as well for a period when my symptoms were at their worst and before treatment. This is an embarrassing area of symptomology to talk about, but it helps to be able to relate to other male patients going through the same things. At least I do have a moderate to good sex drive now, since being on thyroid hormone replacement treatment that is optimal for me.

The same is true of the emotions. They will improve with treatment over time but if you go through an especially bad time with anxiety or depression at some point, don't hesitate to get extra help with that via meds or therapy if you must. It's not something to be ashamed of because you certainly can't help the fact that you have a medical condition going on in your body!

Also be aware that your body may occasionally kick-in with increased symptoms during this process because of medication-dose adjustments and possible thyroid antibody flares on occasion as well (thyroiditis-flares). Antibodies are connected to symptoms because they cause inflammation and can flare up with extra stress or with extra hard physical activity. This aspect is not often mentioned by medical sources, but it is true non-the-less.

The following famous men had/have thyroid disease (mostly the autoimmune type):

* President George Bush Senior

* Bobby Engram, NFL wide receiver with the Seattle Seahawks

* John F. Kennedy Jr. diagnosed (Graves' disease) in 1999

* 2nd Pres. of the U.S. John Adams, is believed to have suffered from Graves' Disease

* Rod Stewart (musician)

* Ben Crenshaw (Pro Golfer)

* Carl Lewis (10 Olympic Gold Medals Track & Field)

Joe Piscipo (actor

* Charles Marion Russell (cowboy artist)

* Roger Ebert (movie critic)

Everything you described to me in your own symptoms, I've been through and I can tell you with absoluteness that it will all improve over time, with your treatment."

7. Stress Management for Thyroid Patients

According to the PubMed medical research article entitled "STRESS AND THYROID AUTOIMMUNITY", stress plays a role in triggering the onset of autoimmune thyroid diseases.

One skill that few people truly possess would have to be successful stress management. Stress seems to play a major role in most of our daily lives, but we can benefit greatly from working on stress management. There are so many ways that stress affects our lives, even in ways that we might not recognize. There are many effective ways to manage it, so that one can begin living a life that is less harmful to their mind, emotions and body.

Stress can continually be a major problem in a person's life especially in these days of living in this crazy, hectic, fast-paced world. Stress can be brought-on and aggravated by many things both major and minor including work, personal life problems, financial issues, relationships, school, children, health problems, or many times from an overload of all these things combined.

Some people even become stressed over the little things such as congested traffic on the road, a long line at the grocery store, house chores and upcoming events or even because a waiter treated them badly at a restaurant. These are just a few examples but there are many other things that cause stress to accumulate in people's lives that can prove to be harmful to them over time.

There are many stress-relievers available for practice to help us deal with the "stressors" of daily life. Yoga and meditation are very popular ways that can help us experience some relief from the stressors of a hectic life. Exercise in general is also a great way to deal with excessive stress. Having an occasional quiet time can also provide some stress reduction, by removing ourselves from everything and everyone for just a few minutes each day. This can help us to calm down and place us back into focus. Deep breathing exercises are another good way to relieve stress, which is simply done by taking, slow, long, deep breaths, inflating your diaphragm, rather than your chest.

Some people suffer stress that is severe enough that they need the help of a therapist to deal with it. This can be a good idea if they are suffering from it severely enough, that they are losing the ability to handle it well on their own.

Hobbies and leisure activities that one enjoys can also be stress relievers. Activities involving art projects, such as painting, drawing, building things, scrapbooking, and gardening are a few simple ways to get one's mind off all the stressors they have been experiencing and to enjoy some leisure time.

8. Treated Hypothyroidism and Weight Gain

It is a well-known fact that untreated hypothyroidism causes moderate weight gain, in fact some patients report weight gain that is in excess of moderate, pre-treatment. I use the term moderate however, because most medical sources state it that way and they also suggest that weight gain with untreated hypothyroidism will usually result in no more than 20lb of weight gain.

Regardless of the actual amount of weight gain that is caused by untreated hypothyroidism, which obviously varies among individual patients and depends on the severity of their untreated hypothyroidism, the fact is that it does cause weight gain! This is since with hypothyroid conditions, the rate of bodily metabolism is slowed down. A hypothyroid person burns less energy when the metabolism is slow and not running at a normal rate. They also refer to this as hypo-metabolism, which can have other causes besides hypothyroidism.

Patients who are being treated for hypothyroidism, still report gaining weight more easily and having difficulty losing weight. There are no medical research studies about weight gain in treated patients, that I am aware of but the number of patients attesting to this problem in articles and forum posts I have been reading since year-2003, is significant. I can personally attest to the fact, that I too gain weight more easily and I have a harder time losing extra pounds, despite being optimally treated for my hypothyroidism.

I'm not sure that we will ever have a firm medical explanation as to why this happens but it could possibly be that thyroid hormone being administered from the outside (hormone replacement therapy), whether it is the natural or synthetic form being prescribed, is slightly less effective in regulating our metabolism than our own naturally occurring hormones are. This is certainly a theory at this point but in my opinion, it is a reasonable one that should be given some consideration by those within the medical profession.

Another theory that I believe should be considered, is the possibility that "thyroid autoimmunity", which is the cause of most cases of hypothyroidism, may also play a factor in weight control. It may be that thyroid antibodies also affect our metabolism, to a small degree but significant-enough to affect our bodily ability to burn calories and to turn fats into energy. It is a fact that "insulin resistance" is more common in treated hypothyroid patients and I can attest I am a hypothyroid patient, who was diagnosed with co-morbid, pre-diabetic insulin resistance.

Treated hypothyroid patients must work harder than people without thyroid disease, to lose weight and to keep their weight under control. While there are many diets plans out there, the same basic principles apply in weight loss, no matter which diet plan you may choose. The principles include eating healthier, which would consist of eating more fruits, vegetables, nuts and grains, cutting back and eliminating refined sugars from your diet, eating less and exercising more. These principles can be wrapped together in many different packages and called by many different diet-plan names, but they are the principles that work, and you simply add discipline to that plan, to make it succeed.

Weight gain and difficulty losing weight is a challenge to treated hypothyroid patients but one they can accomplish with ongoing effort.

9. Doctors Who Test for Thyroid Antibodies

Better qualified Endocrinologists, Thyroid Specialists and other types of MDs who treat thyroid disorders, believe in testing for thyroid antibodies.

Sometime ago, I was talking to a lady, whose husband was suffering symptoms that matched those listed for thyroid disorder, specifically those of "hyperthyroidism" (anxiety, insomnia, weight loss, excessive energy, fatigue etc...). Her husband was tested for his TSH and thyroid hormone levels and the results were within the normal ranges however, the man's TSH was on the increase (his result was above 3.5), according to the new, revised TSH lab standards, set by the AACE (American Association of Clinical Endocrinologists) in the year 2002. The new range set by the AACE for TSH is "0.3 to 3.0". In my discussion with this woman, who was seeking help on behalf of her husband, I told her that her husband's TSH would merit a test of "thyroid antibodies".

Following is what I told her:

"A TSH of "3.58" is not as normal as some Doctors would have you believe. The AACE which is the organization that sets the standard for thyroid testing and treatment, released a new, revised TSH range in late 2002, having "3.0" as the cut off for high normal TSH.

Here's a quote:

"Now the AACE encourages physicians to consider treatment for patients who test outside the boundaries of a narrower margin based on a target TSH level of 0.3 to 3.0." (The AACE)

The National Institutes of Health website states that a person testing with a TSH of above 2.0, should be monitored closely for development of thyroid disease.

Here is a quote:

"Some people with a TSH value over 2.0 mIU/L, who have no signs or symptoms suggestive of an under-active thyroid, may develop hypothyroidism sometime in the future." (NIH/NLM MedLinePlus.com)

My suggestion to you, is to find a qualified thyroid-treating Doctor and get your husband tested for thyroid antibodies. These can reveal thyroid disease going on, in patients with normal-ish hormone levels. The tests are for the "TPO, TG and TSI" antibodies, People with developing autoimmune hypothyroidism (Hashimoto's thyroiditis), can have elevated antibody levels that cause symptoms, even with hormones in normal range. Patients with Hashimoto's thyroiditis (most common cause of hypothyroidism), can go through a period of hyperthyroidism, before the onset of hypothyroidism and the term for this is "Hashitoxicosis".

Here is a quote:

"Hashitoxicosis is an autoimmune thyroid disorder, in which individuals with autoimmune hypothyrodism, usually Hashimoto's thyroiditis (HT), experience intermittent or sporadic periods where they also have symptoms of hyperthyroidism." (Graves' Disease and Hyperthyroidism Wiki)

Amazingly, some Doctors will argue these points, despite the fact that the most reputable medical sources in the world are stating them. Some Doctors believe and state that antibody testing is not necessary unless hormone levels are outside of the normal reference ranges, but the fact is that autoimmune thyroid disease is usually present long before it affects the hormone levels.

This would be my suggestion; to get him tested for "thyroid antibodies". It may confirm or rule out thyroid disease but will be hard to move on to other possible causes of symptoms, if it is not tested for.

Some Doctors jump to snap-diagnoses of emotional problems, such as anxiety and depression, before ordering more complete blood evaluation for patients and to me, this is a dis-service. I believe people with multi-symptom complaints, should not only be tested for thyroid hormone levels and antibodies but should also have a complete blood count (CBC) and glucose levels (A1C) tests, to check for diabetes and other blood disorders.

10. Informational Support for Thyroid Patients

In this article I will list and explain, two major reasons why support and education for thyroid patients is so important.

1. Thyroid patients often express the fact that despite quality treatment for thyroid disease, their doctors do not have time, due to time-constraints, to fully inform them about their thyroid diseases. ---

Most patients feel a great need to understand what is happening to them because the unknown aspects of thyroid disease, can cause them fear and anxiety. This fact certainly doesn't take away from how professional, caring and expert their doctors may be, but the fact is, that there continues to be a growing doctor-shortage in the world. Because of this, doctors simply cannot take the time to thoroughly educate their thyroid patients about the conditions that are causing their thyroid hormone imbalances.

2. Patients experience serious emotional issues from thyroid disease and from the realities of experiencing the onset of a disease that will often affect them, for the rest of their lives. ---

Anxiety and depression are very commonly experienced as "emotional disorders" among treated thyroid patients. A source of support such as a doctor, is not available to a patient throughout the day or night, or at specific times they may be needed to treat emotional flares. Doctors, including those in the psychiatric fields, can only be available to their patients in out-patient settings, for an hour or a few minutes at a time, during office visits. This is comparably very infrequent when considered into daily life. Patients can feel very alone with their disease at times of emotional flares and even those closest to them, may be at a loss for knowing how to support and comfort them.

Consequently, more self-education and support benefits from available resources comes into play (reputable information sources outside of one's doctor but those that he would approve of). The two points expressed above, help to show the purpose for good thyroid disease information and support resources. This includes general information and personal stories, offered by other patients that their fellow-patients can relate to.

It is unfortunate when patients are told that they should not investigate such resources (such as those online) because they "might be led astray with wrong information". It is sometimes implied that they should somehow rely exclusively on their doctors, not only for their essential, prescribed treatments but also for education about their disease and the needed support for coping with it. This simply is not a realistic view and it is not possible in most cases. If a patient's spouse is a doctor or a close relative to them is a medical professional, it might then be possible for them to become self-educated, without relying on reputable outside resources. Also, in the case of a patient who doesn't feel the need for additional education and support, beyond what they receive during doctor visits, they find no necessity for such resources to begin with. For most of us however, we need the additional knowledge and support we find at good information sources, which can actually mean better coping for most of us (and better treatment outcomes, according to medical research conclusions, regarding "proactive patients").

As I have pointed-out, patients should learn from reputable sources and compare/cross-reference information they find, so that it is confirmed as being reliable, by yet other reliable sources. To discourage patients from seeking this type of help, for fear of them being led astray by incorrect information, could mean tremendous lost-opportunities for patients who have serious coping-struggles with thyroid disease.

11. Staying Ready for Thyroid Awareness Month

It always comes back around faster than we realize, so why not stay ready for it ahead of time? January is recognized each year as the month the public is made aware of the importance in monitoring for symptoms of thyroid disease and in seeing their doctor for testing if thyroid dysfunction is suspected (you don't have to wait for January to do that).

The importance in this push each year to make people more aware of thyroid diseases/disorders is in the fact that according to the American Association of Clinical Endocrinologists, half of people who suffer thyroid problems fail to be diagnosed. This is mainly due to their lack of recognition for signs and symptoms of these diseases that affect an estimated 28 million or more (up to 60 million) Americans and a far greater number of people worldwide.

I also feel the importance in Thyroid Awareness Month is in the fact that doctors as well become better-educated in monitoring and testing their patients for thyroid hormone imbalances and "thyroid autoimmunity", which is the class of diseases commonly causing thyroid disorders.

When you consider that tens of millions of people are undiagnosed, it is an incredible realization. Many people suffering symptoms of hypothyroidism for example (under-active thyroid), will believe they are simply stressed out and tired or will attribute symptoms of their slowed metabolism to getting older. People suffering hyperthyroid symptoms (overactive thyroid) will believe they are simply going through an anxious time or are just having a case of nervousness and an unexplained spike in their energy levels. Both conditions also commonly cause goiter (an enlarged thyroid gland) which can also be better recognized with more public education (e.g. learning self-examination of your throat).

Both hypothyroid and hyperthyroid conditions can result in health complications over time if not diagnosed and treated as soon after the onset of them as possible. Both conditions for example can negatively affect the heart over time with hypothyroidism raising cholesterol levels and hyperthyroidism causing hypertension. Both conditions can also affect bone and muscle health due to the weakening of them over time when untreated.

People also commonly experience negative emotional symptoms from thyroid diseases, including anxiety and depression and some patients are recognized by their doctors as having emotional-only problems (something that better education can avoid). These patients may be treated with antidepressants and anti-anxiety medications alone if their doctors do not recognize the need for thyroid function testing and their underlying disease will remain untreated. This can only result in a worsening of their thyroid dysfunction over time.

These are only some of the reasons Thyroid Awareness Month is important, so make sure to tell your family, friends and loved ones to get involved in basic education that will help them recognize when they might be experiencing a thyroid condition. They may also want to learn about common thyroid blood testing, hormone replacement therapy and other drugs for treating thyroid disorders. This can also be done on all other months of the year, besides January.

12. Armour Thyroid Hypothyroid Treatment

How effective is Armour Thyroid hormone medication for hypothyroidism (the brand this author takes)? While very effective in many patients, others may need more T4 hormone added to their therapy.

The purpose of thyroid hormone replacement therapy in treating hypothyroidism, is to replace the low hormone that a person's own thyroid gland is no longer able to produce on its own. The two major thyroid hormones involved in this treatment are the T4 and T3, with T4 being on reserve to be converted in the body into the more powerful T3 (the more metabolically active of the two).

T4 being a "reserve hormone" is how I describe it other articles but it does have a purpose at the tissue level just as T3 does, in regulating bodily metabolism, but only at about 20% compared to T3 (according to medical sources). As a thyroid patient being treated for hypothyroidism with a T4/T3 combination hormone therapy (Armour thyroid brand), I personally want my T3 to be within normal values but not above normal where dose-induced hyperthyroidism is a risk. However, I do not feel as well if mine gets down to mid-range and especially if it is below mid-range (Still within normal but in the lower half, does not work well for me). My doctor works with me in keeping my T3 level as optimal as possible.

It concerned me, when I was first blood retested on Armour Thyroid brand in early 2004 to monitor my thyroid replacement therapy, seeing a low side T4 result, in fact my T3 can be at mid-range and my T4 will actually be flagged slightly low at the same time. I was posting on a MedHelp Thyroid Forum at that time and a Board-Certified MD named Dr. Mark Lupo answers questions there. I asked him about my T4 being flagged slightly low and he said that this was common in patients taking the Armour Thyroid brand for hypothyroid therapy.

Since that time, I've corresponded with and seen the posts of 100s of other Armour Thyroid patients who report that their T4 stays on the low side on Armour as well, even with T3 at good range for them. It made me wonder at times if Armour doesn't have the correct ratio of T4 to T3 for humans. It apparently does however, because the brand has gone through rigorous scrutiny and approval processes via several regulation groups including the USP (United States Pharmacopoeia) and the FDA (Food and Drug Administration).

The T4 to T3 ratio of Armour and other prescribed desiccated T4/T3 brands, is about 4 to 1 (4 times higher in T4). Armour at times, in decades past, has had to recall dose-batches that were found to be inconsistent, but this has not recurred over the past several years. The same thing happened with synthetic T4 brands, including the popular brand "Synthroid" who had recalls of inconsistent dose-batches at times, including a large scale one in 1989. Levothyroxine (levoxyl) brands have had large recalls for inconsistent doses as well, as recently as the year 2002. I mention this to show that Armour Thyroid was not alone regarding past dose recalls.

Some groups say that desiccated T4/T3 drugs like Armour should have a ratio of more T4 in it than it currently has, that would be more like 10 to 1. The manufacturer-Forest Pharmaceuticals however has backing by their medical research representatives, stating that the current 4 to 1 ratio is the most correct one for replacing people with missing hormone in their bodies, due to hypothyroidism. It is an interesting subject and at times I waiver in my own belief on the subject, as to which brands are most reliable because I feel at times that more T4 should be added to the Armour Thyroid brand. I remember reading the testimonials of other patients successfully taking a regimen of Armour, with more T4 added to it (thyroxine added to the dose) and their stories of improvement, are part of what inspired by belief that more T4 is possibly needed than is supplied by an Armour Thyroid dose alone (this may only be true within a certain group/type of patients).

Not only has there been controversy on this issue in the USA but UK groups like "TPA-UK/Thyroid Patient Advocacy" and "The British Thyroid Association" have gone back and forth on this issue, in their debates regarding thyroid hormone brands. At the bottom line, I feel that both in the USA and UK, there is a long way yet to go, regarding more research and trials needed in these areas for the sake of hypothyroid patients, so that there are more definitive answers on these issues for doctors and patients.

13. Selenium for Thyroid Autoimmunity Inflammation

When you have thyroid autoimmunity, including Hashimoto's thyroiditis the most common cause of hypothyroidism, the "thyroid autoimmunity" aspect, can cause illness apart from thyroid hormone levels, according to medical research studies (before hormones become imbalanced or even after they have been corrected). This is a fact that some doctors do not recognize because they are usually of the opinion that until the disease is lowering thyroid hormones to abnormal levels, patients will have no symptoms from the disease. Thyroid autoimmunity causes inflammation within the body, that targets the thyroid gland but that may also have a degree of "systemic effect" (system-wide -- throughout the body). Several studies published by the U.S. National Institutes of Health (PubMed), state this fact. To read an abstract of the study, that cites "endothelial dysfunction" (dysfunction of blood vessels), caused by "Hashimoto's thyroiditis, see the PubMed article titled: "Low-grade systemic inflammation causes endothelial dysfunction in patients with Hashimoto's thyroiditis.", which makes this conclusion.

Also see the research article titled: "Rheumatic manifestations of autoimmune thyroid disease: the other autoimmune disease.", also published at PubMed, for additional interesting-reading on the connection of thyroid autoimmunity, to types of body-wide diseases. These articles can be easily accessed by using their titles as a search-term, in a Google search bar. Thyroid autoimmunity can also cause goiters and nodules in patients who have normal thyroid hormone levels. Some research studies include "anxiety and depressive disorders", as being problems stemming directly from thyroid autoimmunity. The general unwell feeling patients experience with thyroid disease, is in part due to the disease itself. When hormone imbalance also results, this will also contribute to an array of specific hypothyroid symptoms (thyroid hormone deficiency).

Some patients with highly elevated thyroid antibodies, may feel unwell even when they are on proper thyroid dosing, to correct their hypothyroidism (hormone replacement therapy). Some patients with ongoing systemic symptoms, after having their hypothyroidism corrected, may need an anti-inflammatory or supplements like selenium, that help lower the antibodies and their inflammatory effects. Their thyroid medications over time will also help with this task but some patients do not see their thyroid antibody levels lowered to a significant degree, with hormone replacement therapy alone (others may see them significantly lowered). There is patient-individuality involved in this aspect, as with many aspects of autoimmune thyroid disease manifestations.

Also see the PubMed research article titled: "Selenium supplementation in patients with autoimmune thyroiditis decreases thyroid peroxidase antibodies concentrations.", which has a conclusion stating that patients with thyroid autoimmunity, can experience thyroid antibody reductions and reduction in inflammatory activity, by supplementing with selenium.

Thyroid patients who choose to include this over the counter, essential mineral in their treatment regimen, should discuss use of the supplement, with their doctors. They should also follow the manufacturer's instructions on dosing, found on the label of bottles the product is sold in (unless modified by their doctors). Most pharmacies carry the product on their public shelves and it does not require a prescription for use, so it may be worth a trial in autoimmune hypothyroid patients who experience chronic inflammatory types of symptoms, that do not resolve with their hormone replacement therapy.

14. Vitamin D Deficiency and Thyroid Autoimmunity

Vitamin D deficiency has been found in medical research studies, to cause immune system problems and doctors are reporting that deficiencies in the nutrient are becoming more common. There have been studies showing that people with both deficiencies of the vitamin (blood levels of 20 ng/mL and below) and insufficient levels of it (blood-level readings from 30 to 20 ng/mL), are at risk for autoimmune disorders and other chronic and inflammatory diseases, including those affecting the thyroid gland.

My reason for doing research on D deficiency syndromes, is due to my personally being diagnosed with D-deficiency in year 2010 (my blood test result was "17 ng/mL"). I'm currently being treated for this problem and my doctor believes I will require lifelong treatment for it. I have hypothyroidism caused by Hashimoto's thyroiditis and I now have yet another possible cause for mine, being vitamin D deficiency as reported by the conclusions of some medical research study-groups.

Autoimmune thyroiditis very rarely goes into remission or I might should rather say that it rarely ever reverses but it is usually lifelong. While replacing low vitamin D levels is very important, this will not cure the disease. So far, no treatments have been found to cure autoimmunity of any kind, although patients with Graves' disease can see hyperthyroidism permanently resolved with thyroid removal or ablation with radioactive iodine. However, they will afterward have to be treated permanently with thyroid hormone replacement therapy.

One thing that does help to reduce thyroid antibodies (the immune cells that cause the disease) according to other medical research studies, is "supplementing with selenium" at the recommended dose, found on the manufacturer's labels of companies who bottle the nutrient. Other than this, there's no actual cure for thyroid autoimmunity itself. I truly wish there were because I would immediately have the cure administered for mine, if one were discovered and made available. Vitamin D can, however, help to modify/reduce the inflammation aspect of autoimmune diseases and some medical sources recognize the vitamin as a "steroid hormone", in addition to an essential nutrient.

Some sources state that vitamin D deficiency needs to be treated with a "D3" product, rather than with D2, for better improvement. Blood testing sources state that the terms "25-OH vitamin D", "Calcidiol" and "25-hydroxycholecalciferol", are all different names used for the same blood test, that can determine whether a person has adequate or deficient levels of the nutrient within their bodies.

While my own original deficiency reading was "17" as mentioned previously, even a level of 30 is considered "insufficient" and I believe they like to see the level increased to at least 50 or above, for best levels of the nutrient to be available within the body.

15. Basics about Thyroid Cancer

Of all the thyroid disorders and diseases that exist, thyroid cancer is the least common of them all but at the same time is also increasing faster than any other form of cancer. Thyroid cancer should be taken very seriously as should any form of malignancy because any type that is not diagnosed and treated as soon as possible, has the potential to spread to other parts of the body. There are some famous people who have been successfully treated for thyroid cancer, including musician Rod Stewart and comedian/actor Joe Piscipo. Thyroid cancer in fact has a very high treatment success rate and that success rate is increased when early diagnosis and treatment is started.

According to medical research on thyroid cancer, chances of developing it are increased in people with a family history of the disease. It can also be an increased risk in people who are exposed often to radiation in the head and neck areas, such as those who work unprotected around nuclear facilities. Medical researchers also found over 40 years ago that iodine supplementation in people at risk for radiation exposure, can decrease their risk of developing thyroid cancer. Iodine therapy has also been studied and used in some cases of severe thyroid cancer, to slow its progression.

There are five major types of thyroid cancer that include papillary, follicular, medullary, anaplastic and lymphoma. The first two "papillary and follicular" are the most common and medical statistics place these two as accounting for over 90% of cases. Fortunately, they are also the two types that are most successfully treated. The other three types are rare and the "medullary and anaplastic" types are usually more aggressive and can spread rapidly, so patients with these types have a less-favorable prognosis. Thyroid Lymphoma cancer can also grow rapidly but has a higher treatment success rate than do the medullary and anaplastic types.

Thyroid cancers always present as tumors in the thyroid gland, but some tumors are more easily recognizable than others. Some types of tumors take on the appearance of thyroid gland tissue which means they are less malignant and more treatable. The type that resemble thyroid tissue, are referred to as "differentiated". Other types have a distinctly different appearance from normal thyroid tissue and these types are referred to as "undifferentiated" and have a higher malignancy and are more difficult to treat successfully.

There are several procedures used to diagnose thyroid cancer, including blood tests to detect levels of thyroglobulin, cancer cells (new advancements) and for the presence of high "Calcitonin" levels in the blood (found with medullary cancer). Imaging tests may also be ordered, including a Thyroid Ultrasound, CT Scans, MRIs and 24-Hour Thyroid Uptake Scans. The single most diagnostic tests to detect the presence of thyroid cancer, are biopsies of the affected thyroid tissue. This includes using a fine needle to extract tissue samples (Fine Needle Biopsy/Aspiration) and surgical biopsies when needed.

Many thyroid tumors (nodules) are found incidentally, when a person happens to detect one by feel or they may feel a lump on the inside of their throat when swallowing. When a patient sees their doctor, he may also palpate (feel) the nodule with his fingertips, to see if it feels firm or of a significant size. If he finds that the nodule needs further investigation, he may refer the patient for other tests as described above. It bears repeating, to remind of the fact that according to medical sources, only about 5% of thyroid nodules are found to contain cancer.

16. Basics about Thyroid Cancer Treatment

When a patient is confirmed to have thyroid cancer, via medical tests that definitively diagnose it, the treating doctor will refer the patient to a surgeon, who will determine how the cancer will need to be removed. If the cancer affects only one lobe of the thyroid gland (there are two lobes, one on each side), the surgeon may wish to perform what is called a "lobectomy", (partial thyroidectomy) meaning there will be removal of only one side of the gland.

If the surgeon feels removal of only one lobe, still places the patient at risk for the cancer returning, he may instead decide to remove the entire gland, which is referred to as a "total thyroidectomy". The type of surgery that will be performed, is also determined by considering the type of thyroid cancer that is involved. Some types of cancer are more aggressive than others and with these types, the surgeon will always perform total thyroid removal. Surgeons also must determine at what stage the cancer is in -- meaning how far it has progressed.

In order to decrease the risk of the cancer returning, a surgeon may also want to remove the lymph nodes in the neck, that are located near the thyroid gland. These may also be sent off for laboratory analysis to determine if they already contained cancer, which might then lead the surgeon to recommending further treatments.

Additional treatment after any type of thyroidectomy might also include Radioactive Iodine Therapy (RAI) or Chemotherapy, to destroy any remaining thyroid tissue that is capable of absorbing iodine in the body or any remaining cancer cells. Any remaining thyroid tissue that can take up iodine, which is what the thyroid gland is mostly comprised-of, also has the ability to re-develop cancer cells. This is the reason RAI is sometimes used following a Total Thyroidectomy. Chemotherapy is directed at any remaining cancer cells that might remain in the body after a Total Thyroidectomy.

Regardless of the type of thyroid surgery that is performed, thyroid hormone replacement therapy is always used following thyroid cancer surgeries. The goal of the hormone therapy is to suppress the patient's TSH level (pituitary hormone that decreases when thyroid hormone is increased). This also helps prevent recurrence of cancer, but it also replaces any hormone the thyroid gland is no longer capable of producing following surgery. If a patient is given RAI after surgery, they may not be replaced with thyroid hormone for a month or two following the treatment. Most patients will need thyroid hormone replacement therapy following any type of thyroidectomy, as lifelong treatment.

It is very important to see your doctor if you discover any nodules (tumorous growths) on your thyroid gland or if you have difficulty swallowing or feel, that you might have a growth on the inside of your throat. Thyroid cancers have a very high treatment success rate, but that success rate is even higher when thyroid cancers are diagnosed and treated as early as possible.

SECTION FOUR

Autoimmune Aspects of Thyroid Disorders

TABLE OF CONTENTS:

1. Autoimmune Hypothyroid and Hyperthyroid Symptoms

Diseases of thyroid autoimmunity cause both hypothyroid and hyperthyroid conditions to occur. What process is involved, what symptoms result and what are the treatments for autoimmune thyroiditis?

Thyroid autoimmunity is the main cause of both hypothyroid and hyperthyroid cases.

What is Hashimoto's Thyroiditis?

This term simply means that the thyroid glands of affected individuals, are under attack by cells from the immune system, called "thyroid antibodies" (also referred to as "autoantibodies"). These cells are created to eliminate proteins-enzymes within the gland, so that they cannot complete their duties of helping to manufacture thyroid hormones. The two main proteins, also referred to as "globulins", that are being destroyed during thyroid autoimmunity, are the "thyroglobulin" and the "thyroid peroxidase". The names for the antibodies directed against these globulins, are the "Anti-Thyroglobulin" (anti-TG) and the Anti-Thyroid peroxidase" (Anti-TPO). When enough of these have been eradicated by this process, an underactive thyroid gland results, which is referred to as autoimmune hypothyroidism - "Hashimoto's thyroiditis".

Once this process has begun to hinder the manufacture of thyroid hormones enough to slow the affected person's bodily metabolism (the rate of energy produced for the body to function), hypothyroidism sets in. Once it has been diagnosed, the patient's doctor will prescribe a daily dose of thyroid hormone medication, that if taken properly, will restore their metabolism back to within normal values. In many cases, there are several adjustments made to the hormone therapy dose, over several months period, before a patient sees adequate relief of symptoms caused by their lowered metabolism.

The Third Autoantibody Present in Graves' Disease

In the case of autoimmune hyperthyroidism, these same killer cells are present, causing damage to the thyroid gland but an additional antibody called "Thyroid Stimulating Immunoglobulin" (TSI), is also present. This third cell, sent by the immune system, attaches itself to thyroid receptor-cells (TSH receptors), causing excessive production of thyroid hormones. Normally it is TSH that stimulates production of thyroid hormones (Thyroid Stimulating Hormone – from the pituitary gland in the brain). In the case of autoimmune hyperthyroid conditions however, the TSI antibody mimics TSH, so that thyroid hormone production is in-essence being doubled -- with the resulting condition being called "Graves' disease".

In both cases of Hashimoto's thyroiditis and Graves' disease, the anti-TPO and anti-TG, are slowly destroying the thyroid gland but with Graves' disease, the hyperthyroidism can last for an extended period of time (usually years) before the thyroid gland dies-off. Damage to organs and systems of the body will occur if treatment isn't administered, to slow-down thyroid hormone excess. Treatments for Graves' include anti-thyroid drugs which slow hormone production, beta-blocker drugs to address high metabolism symptoms and thyroid gland removal when necessary. The two options for removal of the gland are "thyroidectomy" (surgical) and "Ablation" (a procedure using radioactive iodine to dissolve the gland).

Thyroiditis and Goiters

Both autoimmune hypothyroid and hyperthyroid conditions are considered conditions of "thyroiditis" and can manifest with goiters as a common symptom of them. When the suffix "itis" is added to any term regarding medical terminology, it denotes "inflammation" within the organ or system of the body that is being addressed. With nerve inflammation for example, the term "neuritis" is sometimes used, when a person is experiencing inflamed sinuses, the term "sinusitis" is used and when one refers to thyroid gland inflammation, they should also use the appropriate term, which is "thyroiditis". With any form of thyroiditis, the resulting inflammation can cause the thyroid to swell, which is referred to as "goiter" and this can be true of both Hashimoto's and Graves' diseases. You will note that within the symptom-lists following, that 'goiter' is listed for both conditions of thyroid autoimmunity.

What symptoms prompt testing for thyroid antibodies that cause an underactive thyroid gland?

The following physical signs prompt testing for autoimmune hypothyroidism (Hashimoto's thyroiditis):

- increased sensitivity to cold

- constipation

- dry skin

- puffy face

- hoarse voice

- slowed heart rate (bradycardia – less than 60 beats per minute)

- elevated blood cholesterol

- unexplained weight gain

- muscle aches, tenderness and stiffness

- pain, stiffness or swelling in joints

- muscle weakness

- heavier than normal menstrual periods

- fatigue

- an enlarged thyroid gland (goiter)

- depression

What symptoms prompt testing for thyroid antibodies that cause an overactive thyroid gland?

The following physical signs prompt testing for autoimmune hyperthyroidism (Graves' disease):

- sudden weight loss, even when your appetite and food intake remain normal or increased

- rapid heartbeat (tachycardia – more than 100 beats a minute)

- irregular heartbeat (arrhythmia and skipping beats)

- nervousness, anxiety or panic attacks

- irritability and tremor (fine trembling in your hands and fingers)

- excessive sweating

- changes in menstrual patterns

- increased sensitivity to heat

- changes in bowel patterns, especially more frequent bowel movements

- an enlarged thyroid gland (goiter), swelling appearing at the front base of your neck

- fatigue

- muscle weakness and loss of muscle (atrophy)

- difficulty sleeping

Autoimmune thyroid diseases can develop at any age, but the most common age of onset is between 35 and 40 years of age. Thyroid diseases affect women more commonly than men by approximately an 8 to 1 ratio. Pregnancy also increases the risk for the onset of thyroid disease and so pregnant women need to have their thyroid function tested as well. It is recommended that adults be tested for thyroid disease, beginning at age 35 but they should be tested at any age when hypothyroid or hyperthyroid symptoms appear to be manifesting.

2. Autoimmune Thyroid Disease Basics

Autoimmune thyroid disease is the most common of all autoimmune diseases. Thyroid diseases in general affect an estimated 28-million Americans, 80% of those having the type causing "hypothyroidism", which is five to eight times more common in women than in men (statistics vary).

Most thyroid disorders are caused by autoimmune disease and result in either an under-functioning thyroid (HYPO-thyroidism) or an over-functioning thyroid (HYPER- thyroidism). The symptoms of each of these can be severe and very concerning to the person experiencing them. With hypothyroidism the thyroid gland is slowed down in its ability to produce and distribute "thyroid hormone", which are the cells designed to control the metabolism in our entire body. So, the thyroid in a sense is like a thermostat that regulates the rate at which our bodies operate at. With hyperthyroidism the thyroid gland is sped up, producing and distributing too much thyroid hormone. As stated before, both are most caused by autoimmune disease of the gland.

Autoimmune disease is an improper response by our own immune system because it should normally only direct this response against viruses, allergies, fungus and bacteria but at times, for reasons yet understood by medical science, it will direct this response against normal cells or organs, as if they are one of these intruders/invaders. The immune system does this by sending out killer-cells called "antibodies", that literally attack and kill these unwanted enemies of our bodies. If these antibodies begin attacking an organ, such as the thyroid gland, they will relentlessly do so until they cause damage to the gland and it begins to malfunction. This is the definition of autoimmune disease and it commonly involves the thyroid gland (thyroid autoimmunity).

Many times, during these autoimmune attacks against the thyroid, the gland responds by swelling, as a result from the attack and damage occurring in the gland. This is called a "goiter", meaning a general swelling of the gland from chronic inflammation. Other times the gland will begin developing small tumor-like growths on it, in response to the antibodies attacking, which are called "nodules". Nodules can be "hot" or "cold", meaning they can cause the thyroid to release too much thyroid hormone (hot) or they do not affect hormone production (cold). Hot nodules are seen more often in autoimmune hyperthyroidism, also called "Grave's Disease", while cold nodules are seen more often in autoimmune hypothyroidism, also called "Hashimoto's Autoimmune Thyroiditis".

3. Autoimmunity Challenges of Hypothyroid Treatments

As I begin this chapter, I am reminded of a family member, who repeatedly went to doctors with the full array of hypothyroid symptoms and all of her thyroid hormone levels, including TSH were all within normal range, even with repeated testing. She finally demanded "thyroid antibody tests" and her doctor said, "they were off the map", meaning they were extremely highly elevated, so they opted to place her on thyroid medication because of her symptoms resulting from "thyroid autoimmunity".

Some medical sources state that Hashimoto's thyroiditis (the most common cause of an underactive thyroid) does not cause symptoms, only the resulting hypothyroidism, once detectable by abnormal thyroid hormone blood tests. However, far too many patients report symptoms before hormone levels fall outside of the normal range (abnormally low levels), which also means that the same disease-aspect can continue to cause symptoms when hormone levels are corrected back into the normal range, possibly even at optimal treatment levels.

The description of expected results from thyroid hormone replacement medications, by some sources who state that thyroid autoimmunity is not a factor in symptoms, describe it in almost miraculous or magical terms. One description I read recently, stated to the effect that: "once on thyroid hormone medication, any symptoms a patient has will resolve and they will return to normal within a few weeks". Improvement, yes! Symptoms completely resolved and a return to normal?... No, not in all cases! A percent of patients may see near-perfect results but for many, there is ongoing struggle with a degree of symptoms because autoimmune thyroiditis is a disease and it is not cured by correcting the hypothyroidism that results from it, in fact no cure has yet been discovered (but there is hope of greater improvement with lifestyle changes).

Certainly, we are thankful for the results we do get from hormone replacement therapy but many in the medical community, need to be realistic with patients who can feel let-down by anything less than what they are told will occur with treatment. If perfect relief is not experienced, the patient is told "it is not their thyroid" and in some cases, they will be diagnosed with having psychosomatic/emotional symptoms. Emotional imbalances of depression and/or anxiety may very well be some of the symptoms that do not resolve fully with hypothyroid treatment, but in fairness to the patient, the lack of improvement from adequately/optimally administered hormone therapy, should be described as being "related/attributed" to the thyroid disease (thyroid autoimmunity continues even with corrected hormone deficiencies)..

4. Epstein-Barr Virus and Chronic Disease

With the search/research I've done since my thyroid disease diagnosis in 2003, I am absolutely amazed at how many diseases, especially autoimmune ones, are believed to be directly caused or associated with the "Epstein-Barr Virus" (EBV, EB-Virus). The medical science-research community is taking this virus much more seriously than ever before and many of the most reputable research organizations are suggesting that a vaccine should be developed for this virus because of the potential it has for causing serious diseases. It is also strongly associated with Chronic

Fatigue Syndrome (CFS), according to the Centers for Disease Control, although it may not be a direct cause of the illness.

This virus is far more hazardous to public health than was previously believed for roughly the past 30 years. Medical sources in the past believed that everyone that is infected with EBV becomes immune to it, with no recurrence from it of any kind or complications in it affecting the immune system. There was also previously very little research regarding it causing other diseases but for the past several years, this belief has drastically changed. They now agree that the virus "reactivates" and "replicates" in some people and goes on to cause the development of many other diseases.

The EBV virus is "significantly" more common in autoimmune thyroiditis patients and in Sjogren's Syndrome patients, than in healthy patients, according to the National Institutes of Health/National Library of Medicine (PubMed). You can find this research in the articles they published entitled; "Epstein-Barr virus serology in patients with autoimmune thyroiditis" and "Association of Epstein-Barr virus (EBV) with Sjogren's syndrome: differential EBV expression between epithelial cells and lymphocytes in salivary glands". These articles and those I will refer to following below, can all be found via a simple Google search, using the titles of them as a search term. NOTE: I will be giving summations of these articles in my own words, without making direct quotes from them.

In an article titled; "DIAGNOSTICS AND THERAPY OF EPSTEIN-BARR VIRUS IN AUTOIMMUNE DISORDERS", which is found on the "World Intellectual Property Organization" website, they state that "The Oklahoma Medical Research Foundation", is trying to develop a vaccine for EBV following a filed patent on their proposed idea for one. This firm's research states the fact that a vaccine is needed due to the EBV reactivating in some people, resulting in autoimmune diseases.

In an article found on the "Medical News Today", online magazine, titled; "Epstein-Barr Virus Might Kick-start Multiple Sclerosis" (07 May 2006), they show the association between Multiple Sclerosis and EBV.

In an article on the "Lymphoma Information Network" website, they state that EBV is associated with Hodgkin's Disease and is found present in the blood samples of 40% to 60% of patients with Hodgkin's.

EBV is also common in people with Lupus. It remains dormant or latent in people but can reactivate and becomes a possible trigger for development of Lupus, according to "The Arthritis Foundation", in their article entitled; "Epstein-Barr virus and lupus".

In an article on the "BioMed Central" website titled; "Epstein-Barr virus load in rheumatoid arthritis patients and normal controls: accurate quantification using real time PCR", it states that medical research has identified EBV as a cause of Rheumatoid Arthritis, which they have known for over 20 years.

According to the "Clinical Cancer Research" website, EBV has been implemented as a cause of Burkitt's lymphoma, Hodgkin's disease, non-Hodgkin's lymphoma, nasopharyngeal carcinoma, and lymphomas, as well as leiomyosarcomas, -- some of these, being forms of cancer.

EBV can be a trigger for autoimmune hepatitis, as is discussed in the article found on the "CAT.INIST" website, titled; "Epstein-Barr virus as a trigger for autoimmune hepatitis in susceptible individuals".

Evidence of Epstein-Barr virus affecting mucosal inflammatory cells of ulcerative colitis, is found on the "PubMed" website titled; "Evidence of Epstein-Barr virus infection in ulcerative colitis.".

EBV antibodies are associated with Neurological Diseases, including: Bell's palsy, encephalitis and acute cerebellar ataxia, according to a page on the PubMed website titled; "Epstein-Barr virus antibodies in neurological diseases". They also discuss this in their article titled; "Antibodies to Epstein-Barr virus in neurological diseases", which states that the infected person may have never experienced mononucleosis but is still carrying the EB Virus.

Many of these articles, including the last one I refer to from the PubMed website, clearly state that EBV does not have to become mono at any point to cause these problems and that the virus can "reactivate" and "replicate". This is not hype being published because EBV research is vast and being conducted by ultra-reputable medical research entities. This virus may be one of the most prominent factors in causing autoimmune diseases that is out there. It is incredible that they are just-lately trying to develop a vaccine for EBV. The number of diseases, including autoimmune ones that it is believed to be caused or strongly influenced by EBV, is alarming!

5. Fibromyalgia in Treated Autoimmune Hypothyroidism

Many patients with both hypothyroidism and hyperthyroidism, commonly complain to their doctors about chronic muscle pain. This is a definition of "Fibromyalgia", being co-morbid to thyroid disease (associated with it and possibly stemming from it). It is however, a more common finding in hypothyroid patients, even after they have undergone thyroid hormone correction therapies.

Why would Fibromyalgia Syndrome (FMS) be found to be so common among patients diagnosed with thyroid diseases? According to medical research that has been conducted in this area, which has studied thyroid patients, FMS may be a direct result of "thyroid auto-antibodies". These are the cells produced and sent from the immune system, to eradicate natural proteins and enzymes within the thyroid gland. It is yet to be understood by medical researchers, as to why this occurs. It is evident to them however, that the immune system is recognizing these natural substances that play a factor in the production of thyroid hormones, as enemies to the body. This misguided identification of essential thyroid substances causes damage to the hormone production system, so that hormone-imbalances occur, resulting in either hypothyroidism (an under-active thyroid) or hyperthyroidism (an overactive thyroid).

In hypothyroidism, the two main thyroid proteins that are attacked by autoantibodies, are the "thyroid peroxidase" and the "thyroglobulin". Because of this misguided attack against these proteins, the autoantibodies are referred to as the "anti-thyroid peroxidase" (abbreviated - "TPO") and the "anti-thyroglobulin" (abbreviated "TG"). In the case of hyperthyroid patients (those with "Graves' Disease"), an additional autoantibody will manifest, called "Thyroid Stimulating Immunoglobulin". This later-mentioned immune cell (Abbreviated "TSI"), mimics the action of a pituitary gland hormone called "Thyroid Stimulating Hormone" (TSH). This is what results in the over-production of thyroid hormones or "hyperthyroidism".

Hypothyroid patients on the other hand, will see the TPO and TG auto-antibodies become the predominant ones in their autoimmune thyroid disease, which is referred to as "Hashimoto's thyroiditis". In this case, the immune system attack, renders the thyroid gland unable to produce adequate amounts of thyroid hormones to keep bodily metabolism (cellular energy) at an adequate level. It rather remains at a lower-than-normal level, which is referred to as "hypothyroidism".

Both hyperthyroidism and hypothyroidism have treatments available, to adequately restore bodily metabolism to normal levels. Treatments can accomplish this to optimal levels in some cases (e.g. hyperthyroid patients often have thyroidectomies - surgical thyroid gland removal). The autoantibodies that remain present and that are not eradicated with treatment for hypothyroid patients (treatment consists of thyroid hormone supplementation, rather that thyroidectomy), may result in FMS symptoms. It is not fully understood as to why this is the case, but it is understood that autoantibodies of any kind (in all types of autoimmune diseases), have the potential to cause varied degrees of chronic inflammation within the body. This inflammation from thyroiditis, may prove to be the factor involved in causing FMS symptoms in hypothyroid patients. Medical researchers continue to study this aspect. Hopefully, they will find definitive reasons for the strong association of FMS to autoimmune hypothyroidism, that can remain after treatment of thyroid hormone deficiencies.

6. Hashimoto's Encephalopathy Rare but Serious

There is a neuro-endocrine disorder that causes very serious and potentially life-threatening symptoms, called Hashimoto's Encephalopathy (HE). The disorder can occur in patients with Hashimoto's thyroiditis, who experience a very high elevation of "thyroid antibody" levels. These antibodies, that attack the thyroid gland after recognition of it by the immune system, as a foreign invader, can become highly elevated in these rare cases of HE. At these high elevations they will begin to affect brain and nerve function in the body or the "neurological system". Severe symptoms will result because this system is the body's information and communication center and a disruption from a disease process can cause an array of nerve and brain related symptoms.

Inflammation caused by the antibodies (also called autoantibodies) spreads to the brain and begins to affect the tissue containing the nerves that control bodily functions and impulses throughout the body. The resulting effect, are severe neurological symptoms, meaning abnormal responses and manifestations of nervous system dysfunction. These symptoms can include psychotic episodes (hallucinations and delusions), dementia (mental deterioration), neuropathies (abnormal nerve sensations), seizures and even coma or death if left untreated.

The antibodies responsible for causing thyroid destruction and inflammation in the thyroid gland but that can also cause HE when highly elevated, are the "TPO" (anti-thyroid peroxidase) and "TG" (anti-thyroglobulin) antibodies. This autoimmune process, called Hashimoto's thyroiditis that can result in the less common Hashimoto's Encephalopathy, is more often a result of elevated anti-TPO levels although it can result from elevations of both it and the anti-TG antibodies.

Thyroid hormone levels are not usually a factor in this potentially serious neuro-endocrine disorder of thyroid autoimmunity. Some patients in fact have been documented in medical research, to have experienced HE with their thyroid hormone levels in normal range and before they were in need of thyroid hormone replacement therapy. This disorder is a rare but strong example of the fact that thyroid antibodies can produce bodily symptoms regardless of thyroid hormone levels.

Treatment for HE, is to reduce the inflammation caused by the thyroid antibodies by administering a steroid anti-inflammatory drug to patients who are diagnosed. These drugs, also called corticosteroids or hydrocortisone, mimic the anti-inflammatory properties of our body's own natural anti-inflammatory called "cortisol". A major brand prescribed for inflammatory conditions is "Prednisone", a powerful steroid that usually achieves an anti-inflammatory effect quickly with only a relatively short-term regimen being necessary to correct cases of HE. Patients who are treated, usually see a complete reversal of symptoms and will not experience any long-term complications from HE, once it has been resolved with treatment.

If a patient with Hashimoto's thyroiditis or their loved ones, notice the onset of sudden and severe neurological symptoms, they should report to their Doctor immediately, to rule out HE as the cause. A delay in treatment for a patient experiencing this very rare disorder could result in severe consequences.

7. Inflammatory Symptoms of Hashimoto's Thyroiditis

Published medical research regarding the effects of autoimmune thyroiditis (Hashimoto's disease) contain such phrases as: "systemic inflammatory reaction", caused by this condition, which also leads to hypothyroidism. This means the inflammation is not always localized, within the area of the thyroid gland as some doctors may tell treated hypothyroid patients after they complain of aches and pains and express their suspicions, that their thyroid disease is still causing symptoms. My belief is that some patients have more problems with the inflammatory aspect of their thyroid autoimmunity, than do others.

It is a known fact, that inflammation is a cause of fatigue. It also causes our adrenal glands to remain in overdrive because the "cortisol" hormone, that is produced by them, is not only "the stress hormone" but is also a natural anti-inflammatory agent within the body. It is my feeling as a layperson and an autoimmune thyroid disease patient, that this is why ongoing "fatigued adrenals" can also be a factor in patients with thyroid autoimmunity; a problem that can be addressed and resolved with proper care – (See this site's articles on the subject, under the "Fatigued Adrenals" category).

One of my own treating Endocrinologists, fortunately does-indeed recognize the systemic effect of thyroid inflammation and he stated to me, that this is the cause of my lingering joint pain, that manifested more-so in my shoulders and upper spine, early into my thyroid disease but that is now a body-wide (systemic) problem that I must continue to address. The joint pain resolved at a certain point, early into my hypothyroid treatment and once I had reached an optimal dose of thyroid hormone replacement medication, but it returned approximately 7 years later, to present.

My TG antibodies on an initial thyroid blood panel, showed a result of "537". This was when I was first diagnosed with autoimmune hypothyroidism (normal range <40). In more recent blood retests, these had gone down to "285". This was the point at which my joint pain was near non-existent, but it returned once my antibody levels elevated again, to nearly "400". Is it a coincidence that my symptoms improved, after my antibodies lowered to about half what they were and afterward returned, when they began to chronically increase again? In my opinion, I don't believe so, but I rather think there is a definite correlation between thyroid antibody activity and rheumatic symptoms, in my case.

"Hashitoxicosis" (a condition I experienced short-term) can also be a problem in patients with the type of thyroid autoimmunity that causes Hashimoto's Disease. This medical term simply means that a patient's underactive thyroid will surge occasionally, with extra release of hormone, causing phases of hyperthyroidism and then settles back down into a hypothyroid or euthroid state afterward. This can cause an array of hyperthyroid symptoms but is something you seldom hear doctors talk about because as with many things of this type, they believe the problem is "very rare", when it may actually be common in milder forms. Some doctors also state that sub-clinical adrenal insufficiency (Adrenal Fatigue) is "very rare" in thyroid patients and that emotional symptoms and joint pain are also rare, if a patient's thyroid hormones are within normal range (after correction of their hypothyroidism).

However, large numbers of patients are complaining of these symptom-problems from highly elevated antibody levels, despite being on adequate or optimal hormone replacement treatment. There simply cannot be this many "psychosomatic" thyroid disease patients out there! If the related medical research that has been conducted in this area is correct, then we can conclude that the reason for symptoms in many of these patients, is a result of inflammation from thyroid autoimmunity and not from imbalances of thyroid hormone levels alone.

8. Mixed Hypothyroidism with Hyperthyroidism

Most people with hyperthyroid (overactive) or hypothyroid (under-active) thyroid glands have "thyroid autoimmunity" as the cause. I'll first mention some basic things about the two disorders of thyroid hormone imbalance but will also add some not-too-often recognized facts on the close relationship of Hashimoto's thyroiditis to Graves' Disease, following below.

When hypothyroidism occurs from antibodies attacking the thyroid gland, it is referred to as "Hashimoto's thyroiditis". There are other types of chronic thyroiditis that are like Hashimoto's, but these are rare, and doctors usually place them under the 'Hashimoto's umbrella' if they are chronic (ongoing/permanent types that lead to hypothyroidism).

Alternatively, when hyperthyroidism occurs from antibodies attacking and attaching to the thyroid gland, it's called "Graves' disease" (another term is "Toxic Diffuse Goiter").

Some hypothyroid patients essentially have both diseases at certain early points after the development of thyroid autoimmunity, but this usually happens as a temporary thing, referred to this as "Hashitoxicosis". Uncommonly it can be a permanent wavering back and forth between the two types of hormone imbalances and when this happens even doctors can be stumped as to whether a case falls within the Hashimoto's or Graves' category.

It's not recognized as being common but I have personally read emails and I have seen posts by people on thyroid forums, who are affected by this mixed-condition, which means that it does happen to a percent of thyroid patients. It's possible that "Chronic Hashitoxicosis" (a permanent mix of Graves' and Hashimoto's) is not as rare or near non-existent as was once believed and that some doctors may not be recognizing it in their patients who manifest with it.

A treatment that has been used in parts of Europe for mixed thyroid disease, as described above, is something called "block & replace therapy". They administer this treatment by giving patients a regimen of a high-dose anti-thyroid drug to slow thyroid hormone production and at the same time, or in an alternating fashion, they will replace the resulting low thyroid hormone (hypothyroidism), with a second drug. This treatment is rare in the U.S. but may become used more-commonly over time (purely speculative). There are no statistics available in regard to how successful this treatment is in patients with mixed thyroid disease, but it may be an option to consider in hypothyroid patients, who appear to be candidates for thyroidectomies, meaning surgical removal of their thyroid glands.

9. Permanent versus Temporary Thyroiditis

In corresponding with a number of autoimmune hypothyroid patients, also termed as having "Hashimoto's Thyroiditis", they have reported being told by their doctors, that their hypothyroid condition is "just a temporary case of thyroiditis" and that it should resolve in a relatively short period of time. I was also told this by a doctor during an office visit, who was listed as an Endocrinologist. He was reviewing my blood test results, showing both TPO (anti-Thyroid Peroxidase) and TG (anti-Thyroglobulin) antibodies being highly elevated and my thyroid hormone levels being below normal, "hypothyroid" (a clear indication of permanent thyroiditis).

I had done just enough research at that time, to know that elevated antibodies, that had been present long enough to begin lowering my thyroid hormone levels, was not a temporary condition, that would resolve over time! Once the thyroid begins to under-function due to damage from an attack by autoantibodies, it cannot be reversed and the patient will have to begin thyroid hormone replacement medication, that will most likely remain a lifelong treatment. In very rare cases, Hashimoto's will reverse, and the antibodies will diminish, before permanent damage to the thyroid has occurred (very rare). For most Hashimoto's patients, the autoimmune process continues to damage the thyroid, eventually resulting in the need for permanent hormone replacement therapy. The point being, that Hashimoto's is not a temporary form of Thyroiditis but a chronic, permanent form.

There is a temporary form of thyroid gland inflammation, called "Sub-acute Thyroiditis", "deQuervain's Thyroiditis" and "Viral Thyroiditis" (each referring to the same or very similar condition). This is very likely the type of transient thyroiditis doctors are referring to and that they may mistakenly believe Hashimoto's patients are experiencing. Most of these transient types are much rarer than Hashimoto's thyroiditis and they have characteristics that differentiate them from permanent thyroid autoimmunity. Another type of temporary thyroid inflammation, is "Silent Thyroiditis", which occurs in from 5 to 10 percent of women, post-partum, which makes it a more common type but the requirement for it to take place after giving birth, gives it a very distinct diagnostic criteria.

The confusion between Sub-acute Thyroiditis and Hashimoto's, may be in doctors seeing elevated thyroid antibody levels on patient's blood lab results. According to medical resources however, Sub-acute Thyroiditis, usually causes only mild elevation of thyroid antibodies and in most cases, no elevation of them at all. This temporary form of thyroid inflammation also only lasts approximately four weeks, before it completely resolves. The major symptom with the temporary form of thyroiditis, is rapid onset of severe pain and inflammation, in the thyroid area. This sudden onset, in most cases will cause "hyperthyroidism" and not "hypothyroidism". When an underactive thyroid does result from the transient type, it is usually mild and temporary. This means patients will usually complain of hyperthyroid symptoms such as nervousness and sweating, rather than noticing any hypothyroid ones, when temporary thyroiditis occurs (e.g. constipation and feeling cold).

While Hashimoto's Thyroiditis, is an autoimmune disease, Sub-acute Thyroiditis, is often caused by a viral infection, such as "Mumps" or "Upper-respiratory Infections ", that settle into the thyroid gland. With Hashimoto's, patients will have elevated antibodies against the thyroid gland itself, while with Sub-acute Thyroiditis, patients will have elevated antibodies against the virus causing the thyroiditis. To add to the occasional confusion, Hashimoto's patients at times, will have attacks of thyroiditis but this does not take away from the fact that they also have autoimmune disease as the root cause of their thyroid condition and the thyroiditis flares, are only a feature of it (this does not occur in all Hashimoto's patients).

To sum up the differences, if a patient does not complain of severe pain in the thyroid gland area and they have highly elevated thyroid antibody levels, it is most likely Hashimoto's Thyroiditis and not Sub-acute Thyroiditis. Also, if the condition is ongoing for more than a few weeks, this should also reveal to the patient and doctor, that it is permanent rather than temporary form of thyroiditis.

10. Recognizing Graves' Disease - Hyperthyroidism

Some statistics estimate that over three million Americans suffer from Graves' disease. This thyroid disorder that causes hyperthyroidism (over-active thyroid), is caused by an autoimmune response that sends out antibodies to attack the thyroid gland.

Graves' disease results in a type of hyperthyroidism, caused by an autoimmune response in the body. With Graves' disease, a patient will have antibodies sent out by the immune system to attack their thyroid gland. Some of these antibodies also attach to the thyroid gland and in response, the gland produces more thyroid hormone and the levels become too high for the body's metabolism to function properly. The sped-up metabolism is called "hyperthyroidism" and Graves' disease is the most common cause of an over-functioning thyroid gland (up to 95% of cases).

The main antibody that cause Graves' disease is called "thyroid stimulating immunoglobulin" (TSI). Patients who develop Graves' disease can have several antibodies directed against their thyroid glands, including the "anti-TPO" and the "anti-TG". These antibodies cause destruction of the gland, plus swelling and goiter from resulting inflammation. The type of antibody that contributes to the hyper-functioning of the gland, however, is the TSI antibody, as previously mentioned. These are the ones that help to better diagnose a hyperthyroid patient as having Graves' disease; TSI antibodies are detected in a patient using blood lab testing.

Graves' disease patients can develop nodules on their thyroid glands that contribute to the over-production of thyroid hormone. These nodules are small tumors that begin to develop within the thyroid gland and some of these are what are referred to as "hot nodules", meaning they cause an increase in thyroid hormone production. Not all nodules that develop in a diseased gland become "hot"; many do not cause the thyroid to become stimulated to over-produce and these are referred to as "cold nodules". Some patients who have multiple nodules that are hot are termed as having a "toxic nodular goiter". If a patient simply has thyroid enlargement or goiter that is characteristic of the disease, it is referred to as "diffuse toxic goiter", which is also another term for Graves' disease. The symptoms of Graves' disease are those of a sped-up metabolism. A person with hyperthyroidism, caused by Graves' disease, may experience the following symptoms: anxiety, nervousness, weight loss, diarrhea, sweating, oily skin, depression, goiter, rapid heart rate, hypertension, muscle weakness, tremor, hair loss, bone degeneration and increased appetite.

If not treated, patients with Graves' disease have increased risk for serious health problems. The disease must be diagnosed and treated if a patient is suspected of having it because if left untreated, problems can develop including heart disease, organ damage from hypertension, chronic osteoporosis and Graves' Ophthalmopathy (GO), which is an inflammatory problem affecting the eyes. This eye disorder, also called "thyroid eye disease" (TED) can cause serious damage and even blindness in some patients. Unfortunately, regarding Graves' disease, patients who do develop GO may not be able to prevent some degree of eye damage even though they are well treated for their hyperthyroidism.

People with hyperthyroid symptoms need to see a licensed physician to have proper testing and diagnosis of the cause for their symptoms. If Graves' disease is diagnosed as the cause, there are effective treatments to help correct symptoms and any resulting complications.

11. Thyroid Disease Antibodies

Most patients with both hypothyroidism (underactive thyroid) and hyperthyroidism (overactive thyroid) are experiencing autoimmune diseases that cause these conditions. When autoimmune thyroid disease results in hypothyroidism, the term for the disease is "Hashimoto's thyroiditis." When the autoimmune disease of the thyroid causes hyperthyroidism, it is called "Graves' Disease." The paragraphs below help to bring better understanding to the subject of "thyroid antibodies."

"Thyroid antibodies" are what cause "autoimmune thyroid disease" in patients who develop them. The immune system normally sends out antibodies, which are killer cells, to eradicate foreign invaders from the body that can make us sick. These invaders include viruses, bacteria and allergens. The purpose of antibodies is to seek these-out and destroy them, to prevent our bodies from becoming ill. The problem with "thyroid antibodies" in the case of hypothyroidism (80% of cases), is that, like other antibodies that cause autoimmune diseases, they are directed against the thyroid gland as if it is one of these invaders. It is a case of mistaken identity that over time causes damage to the thyroid gland and cell death. Eventually, the antibodies will kill-out the thyroid gland completely (resulting in overt hypothyroidism).

The types of antibodies that cause an under-functioning thyroid from Hashimoto's thyroiditis, relentlessly attack the gland, until it becomes damaged and unable to function at its original level. Once enough damage has been done to the gland and a significant percent of thyroid cells have been killed, the onset of hypothyroidism occurs. The low level of functioning will usually be mild at first (sub-clinical) and over time will worsen, unless the patient with hypothyroid autoimmunity receives treatment. The opposite is true of patients with Graves' Disease because in their case, the antibodies directed against the thyroid gland, stimulate it to produce excessive amounts of thyroid hormone or a what is also called an over-functioning thyroid gland.

What are the names of the main antibodies tested for in these two types of autoimmune thyroid diseases? In Hashimoto's Disease, the two main antibodies that cause thyroid gland destruction and resulting hypothyroidism are the anti-Thyroid Peroxidase Antibodies (abbreviated TPO) and the anti-Thyroglobulin Antibodies (abbreviated TG). In Grave's

Disease, the main antibody that causes stimulation of the thyroid gland to produce too much hormone is called Thyroid Stimulating Immunoglobulin (abbreviated TSI). These antibodies (for both diseases) are detected by means of blood lab tests.

12. Book Review For – Hypothyroidism in Childhood and Adulthood

This review is for a book that is an asset to thyroid patient advocacy. The two women who authored it, have done a superb job relating their history of hypothyroid treatment failures and successes.

This wonderful book is available, about hypothyroidism by C Phillips and D Roach -- twin sisters who developed hypothyroidism during childhood and who have now entered the age of their 40s (born in 1968). The book is titled "Hypothyroidism in Childhood and Adulthood". These two women have kept diaries since youth, detailing their treatments for hypothyroidism, via "T4 only", "T3 only" and "T4/T3 combo", thyroid hormone therapies. In my opinion, the information they provide in this written work, should be used by medical research groups, as a study for improving thyroid hormone replacement therapy for hypothyroid patients, including that which is administered to both youths and adults.

An Explanation for What T4 and T3 Hormone Medications Actually Are

For those reading this book review, who do not understand what "T4" hormone therapy is for example, this simply represents the type of hormone that is used to treat a patient's hypothyroidism. Actually, "T4 only" thyroid hormone replacement, is the most prescribed for hypothyroid patients, to replace their low thyroid hormone levels. The brand that is usually prescribed in the USA, is the "Synthroid®" brand but in the UK, they usually call their T4 brand by the name "Levothyroxine", which comes in brand names such as "Eltroxin", among others.

Both medications are basically the same -- they are synthetic T4 hormone preparations, that are prescribed by doctors to treat hypothyroid patients. The "T4" means that it is a thyroid hormone containing 4 iodine molecules. When "T3" is referred to, this means it is a hormone preparation containing 3 iodine molecules. Doctors will at times, prescribe T3 only drugs to treat people with underactive thyroid glands.

Debates Continue Over Which Thyroid Hormone Therapy is Superior

There has been ongoing debate for many years, as to which prescribed thyroid hormone preparation is best for treating hypothyroidism. Since the thyroid gland naturally produces both T4 and T3, many advocates for brands containing both, such as the "Armour® Thyroid" brand, believe that best results for correcting hypothyroidism, can only be accomplished by taking this brand. When T4 only is prescribed to a patient with hypothyroidism, the doctor and patient, are depending on a conversion process to occur within the body, in which the T4 will convert into any T3 that is needed in the body (the conversion process occurs mainly within the liver).

Some Doctors are Not Updated Regarding Best Hypothyroid Treatments

So, to sum up the different treatment options that doctors may prescribe, there is T4 only, T3 only and combination T4/T3 thyroid hormone preparations that may be prescribed. Much of what determines which type/brand a doctor prescribes, has to do with the history of how well patients have responded to treatments. Unfortunately, there are doctors who are less-specialized in the area of thyroid treatments and who are not updated as well as they should be, regarding successful trends within the medical community and they will under-treat their patients, leaving them in a perpetual state of subclinical hypothyroidism.

Within this book I am reviewing, the two women-authors, relate their hypothyroid treatment experiences, with each of these types of thyroid hormone preparations, prescribed to them by different doctors during their childhoods, young adults years and now as they have entered middle age. It seems evident by their life stories as thyroid patients, that some doctors who treated them, were more highly specialized and updated than were the others. I am grateful for their providing me a free review copy and I sincerely hope to do justice in relating my experience with reading this revealing, written work, that I believe to be an important asset to "thyroid patient advocacy".

Fixing Hypothyroid Treatment that is Already Working Perfectly

When these women were young girls, they were diagnosed with hypothyroidism and were treated by a pediatrician with synthetic T4 hormone replacement and dosed with the medication, to suppress their elevated TSH levels. Thyroid Stimulating Hormone (TSH) is the pituitary hormone that reflects thyroid hormone levels and decreases to a lower level when thyroid hormone levels increase in the body. Their treatment as youths placed their TSH levels at undetectable levels but at the same time, greatly relieved their hypothyroid symptoms. This is supposed to be the goal of hypothyroid treatment however, during a blood retest of their TSH, by a new treating doctor (a general practitioner), he decided to reduce their dose out of fear that their suppressed TSH levels presented with the possibility that they would experience osteoporosis (a danger from over-treatment with thyroid hormones). This dose change at youth, caused them to spiral down again into hypothyroid symptoms. It also began an incredible journey for both girls, to find a thyroid hormone therapy that would gain them back, an improved quality of life.

Symptoms of Inadequate Treatment, Return with a Vengeance

Following a dose decrease as suggested by the GP, they fell into severe hypothyroid symptoms but were told incorrectly, that the symptoms were from the need for the dose decrease that was given just in time. When the symptoms were not relieved after several months however, the girls insisted upon reevaluation of their treatment. Their symptoms had become so severe as to make them disabled and also required that they see other specialized doctors for severe joint pain (mainly in their arms, hands and backs). A new private doctor they were referred to at one point increased their thyroxine/T4 dose but the increase was still below the dose that brought them much better symptom relief, when they were smaller children under the pediatrician's care, who first treated them optimally.

The Girls are Given a Trial of T3 Only Hormone Therapy

Their doses were eventually returned to that original best-level that brought them the most improvement in hypothyroidism. However, unlike the results they had at their earlier ages, when under the care of the pediatrician, they did not experience significant symptom relief of their hypothyroidism although they were much improved. Their newer treating doctor began a trial of T3 therapy (triiodothyronine), added to their T4 and began to wean them off the T4, eventually replacing them with T3 only. The girls again experienced a significant degree of symptom-relief but were still in need of much more improvement from their hypothyroid symptoms.

As Young Women, the Twins were Placed on Natural T4/T3 Combination Hormone Therapy

The girls who had now become women, were eventually administered a combination T3 and T4, hormone replacement medication, porcine derived (processed pig thyroid glands), called "Armour® Thyroid". This is in fact the brand of thyroid medication I, the author take and they saw the most significant relief of their hypothyroid symptoms since childhood. It is my take from the final chapters of their book that they still have room for improvement, but they have regained much of the activities important to life, that they were once disabled from participating in. Both of them have also achieved bachelor's Degrees of Science and are now better-able to attend family events and live more satisfying lives since experiencing their much-needed improvement. It is simply a fact that some patients see more improvement on T3/T4 combination hormone therapy and this book is another confirmation of that fact.

An Interesting Case Study on Hypothyroid Treatments

This book is greatly interesting, and the ladies have photographs included in the book, showing the differences between the two girls, when one of them first experienced hypothyroidism, before the other one did. The stunted growth this caused in the twin that first became ill is remarkable, but this same twin caught up with her sister in development, once treated with thyroid hormone therapy. They also include symptom and lab test graphs that detail their treatments over the years.

Hypothyroid Treatment Should Be Based on Symptom Relief as well as TSH Levels

I commend these women for a book that so intelligently details the treatment of their hypothyroidism and how they detail much of this in a medical study type format. I feel the important message this book sends, includes the importance in doctors not treating patients using the TSH-only test (full thyroid panels can better reveal hormone therapy results). I also believe it conveys the importance in doctors not overreacting to possibilities such as the development of osteoporosis from over-treatment because this possible complication can also be monitored (as it was in their case) using lab testing as well. If patients are experiencing significant symptom-relief, their thyroid hormone dose should not be adjusted with decreases, unless absolute proof of over-treatment is presented. Radical dose changes can cause an imbalance that is ongoing and not easily correctable, as the story of these two ladies, so adequately demonstrates.

This book is a great read for thyroid patients and doctors alike!

SECTION FIVE

Anxiety and Depression in Thyroid Disorders

TABLE OF CONTENTS:

1. Antidepressants Combined with Thyroid Hormones

Several times over the past few years, SSRI Antidepressants have been the subject of discussion on thyroid forums where I have posted-on or where I have been moderator. I also receive occasional emails from thyroid patients asking questions about these drugs regarding their effect on thyroid hormones in the body.

These drugs prompted one of my first-ever searches online because as a newly diagnosed hypothyroid patient in early 2003, I was also prescribed an SSRI antidepressant. I was curious as to how these drugs might affect my thyroid hormone treatment. In my case I ended up weaning-off the drug because my doctor at the time, in my opinion was acting too-quickly in prescribing the long-term drug, by not first allowing my thyroid hormone replacement therapy to relieve my symptoms of increased anxiety and intermittent low mood.

In my case, my hypothyroid therapy alone, did very well in balancing my depressive emotions and I was not in need of an SSRI antidepressant for this. I did continue to experience aspects of anxiety disorder, which continues to affect me presently. Mine, however, is a lifetime anxiety condition that does not respond well to antidepressants and I have been dealing with the disorder since my youth -- long before I was diagnosed with thyroid disease.

I did see my anxiety symptoms increase greatly, during a phase of "Hashitoxicosis" that my autoimmune hypothyroidism, first manifested with in year-2003 (transient/temporary hyperthyroidism). It was as if I was experiencing a continuous panic attack during this phase, but the panic symptoms subsided, when the Hashitoxicosis ended. Following this phase, I began to experience progressive, lifetime hypothyroidism, for which I am now well-treated. In short, I am a hypothyroid patient, who does not do well taking SSRI antidepressants. Other treated hypothyroid patients I have known, do very well on the drugs and benefit greatly from them.

Medical research has been conducted, regarding antidepressants and their effects on thyroid hormone. Let me again express the fact, before I mention more about these studies, that I'm a firm believer in the ability of these drugs to be extremely effective in people who need them. I do feel however that there is an area of education about these drugs that thyroid patients should be given (or that they should obtain through careful online search), especially if the drug is added by their doctor to their hypothyroid, hormone replacement therapy.

It's possible, according to research I have studies on reputable medical sites, such as the U.S. National Institutes of Health ("PubMed"), that some patients will either need their hormone dose adjusted due to the slight lowering-effect the drugs have on thyroid hormones or they might need the addition of "T3" to their hormone replacement therapy (most doctors treat with T4 only), if T3 is not already in their treatment regimen.

Studies published by the U.S. National Institutes of Health state that SSRI antidepressants have been found to lower thyroid hormones in the body, to some degree. One of these is titled "Peripheral thyroid hormones and response to selective serotonin reuptake inhibitors". You can read the abstract study by using this title in a Google search. There is also a PubMed article citing studies regarding better improvement in treated hypothyroid patients, placed on SSRI antidepressants when T3 is added to their hormone therapy. A Google search using this medical study title: "T3 augmentation of SSRI resistant depression.", will provide a reader the link to this abstract article.

The first research article I refer to by title above, doesn't specifically refer to the lowering of thyroid hormone as "thyroid dysfunction", in patients who are prescribed SSRI antidepressants. However, you could still say that the drugs can hinder thyroid hormone levels enough in some patients, as to merit use of increased thyroid hormone replacement to supplement the SSRI therapy (a recommendation stated within the second study I give title for, above). I believe these facts point to the need for better public education on this subject and for improved doctor-patient communication regarding SSRI drugs, prescribed to thyroid patients taking hormone replacement therapies.

The important thing for patients who have these drugs added to their thyroid hormone therapies, in addition to monitoring for possible side effects, is to ask their doctors to order "thyroid panel blood tests" within a few weeks of combining them. This is to see how their hormone levels are affected and if it might result in the need for them to be given a dose-increase of T4 and/or T3, should either or both become lowered by the SSRI antidepressant medication. This would be more of a concern for those patients and doctors, who wish to see thyroid hormone therapies, optimized to the best levels possible.

2. Anxiety Attacks in Hashimotos Thyroiditis Patients

Hypothyroidism related anxiety, is a subject I've addressed in other articles and the number of e-mails I get from patients who suffer anxiety from their hypothyroidism, especially the newer diagnosed patients with "Hashimoto's thyroiditis" as the cause, is the highest percent of any I receive. Anxiety with hypothyroidism, is also a very common subject on thyroid disease forums as well.

Below, is a response I made to a longtime friend of mine who wrote me some time ago with a question on this very subject. I mention to her in my response, that in some cases the anxiety symptoms that hypothyroid patients experience, is caused by a condition called "Hashitoxicosis". (Note: In a Subsequent email, she stated that her hypothyroidism was caused by Hashimoto's thyroiditis.)

My reply:

"I would almost bet your hypothyroidism is caused by "Hashimoto's thyroiditis" because it is the autoimmune type and by far the most common cause. It is confirmed by positive blood tests of "thyroid antibodies". These are the "anti-TPO and anti-TG" antibodies and these are what attack a person's thyroid and kill off its cells over time. The immune system mistakenly recognizes your thyroid as an invader, like it does with viruses, allergens and bacteria.

With Hashimoto's, you can go through a period of "Hashitoxicosis" (actual medical term), especially early into the onset of hypothyroidism that it causes because the thyroid will waiver back and forth between producing low hormone and having surges of increased hormone, as it tries to avoid hypothyroidism and spurts back to life. This is a real condition and I've seen the testimonies of literally 100s of patients who experience panic attacks from it and I am one who also experienced this condition, when I was newly diagnosed. Some medical sources state that Hashitoxicosis is rare, while I believe it is likely more common in milder forms.

Strangely doctors sometimes do not seem to know about this condition that goes with autoimmune hypothyroidism. They may tell patients their anxiety is not caused by their diagnosed thyroid disease but that it is a separate issue. Many times, they will prescribe additional medications for it, before giving thyroid hormone replacement medication a chance to work.

There is a Dr. Richard Hall MD, also a professor of psychiatry who has been involved in research studies at major medical universities, such as John Hopkins University and in his studies on the relationship of anxiety to endocrine disorders, it was found that in patients with "Hashimoto's thyroiditis", anxiety was a common symptom at the time patients were diagnosed.

There are also studies that have been published on the "PubMed" website, which is provided by The National Institutes of Health and The National Library of Medicine, stating that anxiety symptoms and anxiety disorders are associated with Hashimoto's disease, which is also the most common cause of hypothyroidism in industrialized nations.

Doctors often do not recognize Hashitoxicosis, unless full blown symptoms of transient hyperthyroidism are occurring (a temporary phase of it). One wonders however, if the fluctuations that Hashimoto's-hypothyroid patients have commonly in their thyroid hormone levels, is not also a mild manifestation of Hashitoxicosis, even if full-blown phases of hyperthyroidism do not occur? What if upward, temporary increases in their thyroid hormones, only cause them "increased anxiety" as a symptom, rather than a full array of hyperthyroid symptoms? If this cannot be recognized as Hashitoxicosis, then why not classify it as something like "Mild Hashitoxicosis" or "Thyroiditis Flares"?

These are the questions I have as a treated hypothyroid patient, who is attempting to help bring general information to fellow patients. In the meantime, we are truly grateful for the medical research that continues to be undertaken on thyroid disease subjects and we eagerly await further developments and the better-defining of terms describing autoimmune hypothyroid disease manifestations."

3. PART A: Anxiety Catastrophic Thinking in Thyroid Patients

What are "catastrophic thoughts" and why do they occur in people with chronic anxiety disorders? Can this phenomenon of "what if" thinking be reversed or halted, to improve their quality of life Catastrophic thoughts can occur with any anxiety disorder, although it is more common in people suffering from "Generalized Anxiety Disorder" (chronic free-floating anxiety) and in those with "Panic Disorder" (frequent panic attacks).

Catastrophic Thoughts

This type of thinking usually involves thoughts that an anxiety sufferer finds to be distressing and bizarre. Many times, the thoughts include their fear of "acting out" in such ways that are not characteristic of them. They might for example have thoughts stemming from the fear that their anxiety will cause them to lose control and to act crazy in front of onlookers. Other sufferers might have thoughts of passing out from an anxiety attack and not being somewhere when this feared event occurs, in which medical help can arrive, to revive them.

One area of catastrophic thinking that can be especially concerning to an anxiety disorder sufferer, are those thoughts in which they fear becoming violent to others around them, such as family members or their own children. The fact is however, that all of these types of feared catastrophes, are irrational in the vast number of cases and have an extremely low possibility of ever taking place. These types of thoughts are, however, very common to people suffering disorders of chronic anxiousness and they often find that their enjoyment in life is seriously hindered by them. When these thinking patterns are recognized, it is time for the affected person to seek ways to reverse them or to even halt them from taking place, so that they can restore to themselves, a better quality of life.

Treating "What If" Thinking

One very effective method for overcoming catastrophic thoughts, is simply to recognize that they are irrational and that they will not take place. This is an aspect of "Cognitive Behavioral Therapy" (CBT), that is taught to anxiety disorder sufferers. What a mental health therapist will usually do, in beginning this method, is to explain to an anxiety sufferer, that the thoughts occurring to them, are actually a result of a very natural mechanism within the body called "the fight or flight response". This built-in anxiety reaction is supposed to occur when we become threatened, however, in anxiety disorders it occurs "out of context" and with an abnormally high frequency (more often than it should). It is not the mechanism that is unnatural but only the timing of it, and frequency of it that is disordered. The mind at times that this response is activated, begins to scan for every possible danger. Therefore, the mind begins to consider every possibility of danger, hence -- catastrophic thoughts will begin to flood the mind.

Replacing Negative Thoughts

Sufferers of chronic anxiousness should understand that by the very fact of catastrophic thoughts being unpleasant to them, this means that they will not act on them and cause them to transpire. Only when a person takes pleasure in the thought of acting out some bizarre behavior, is there any danger that they will do so. In addition to anxiety sufferers being taught about the fight or flight response, during CBT therapies, they will also be taught methods for replacing their bizarre, fearful thoughts, with those that are positive and calming. This may include thinking about their family or about leisure activities or hobbies they enjoy. Some patients may learn to inject humor into their catastrophic thoughts, which can help to reverse them or to halt them completely.

Anything that can be used to divert negative thoughts, toward positive ones, is acceptable and should be practiced by anxiety disorder sufferers who want to conquer these undesirable thought-processes in their lives.

PART B: Anxiety Catastrophic Thinking in Thyroid Patients

Catastrophic thinking is an extremely unpleasant anxiety disorder aspect, but sufferers can learn to defeat it. Diversionary thoughts can stop irrational, fearful thinking, with time and practice. To recap what was discussed in "PART A" of this article, A catastrophic thought, would simply be one that ponders the possibility of the most undesirable outcomes for any given situation. When a person practices these type thoughts, on a frequent basis, they become "catastrophic thinkers".

What Kinds of Thoughts Do Catastrophic Thinkers Have Specifically?

People who develop chronic, irrational thinking, not only expect the worst outcomes for things they are involved with in real time but they usually also think about horrible things happening in the future, even when there is no real scenario or basis for them to occur (irrational). This is most often a manifestation of chronic anxiety -- a symptom-aspect that can occur with every type of disorder, involving severe anxiousness.

Following are examples of catastrophic thinking, that can occur with the different types of anxiety and stress disorders:

•	Post-Traumatic Stress Disorder – A fear that past traumatizing event(s), will recur

•	Panic Disorder – A fear that future panic attacks will cause sudden death or insanity

•	Social Anxiety Disorder – A fear that one will be judged as a fool or hated by others

•	Generalized Anxiety Disorder – A fear that things of personal importance will fail miserably, become damaged, injured, destroyed or permanently taken away

•	Agoraphobia – A fear that horrible, immediate dangers to body and emotions, exist everywhere outside of the home

These are just some of the general areas of phobic thinking that can occur within the minds of anxiety sufferers.

Scanning for Possible Dangers that are Highly Improbable

When chronic anxiousness or panic is experienced by someone, this means that the "fight or flight response" is activated, which causes the mind to scan for any possible dangers. This is the reason bizarre thoughts will enter the minds of anxiety disorder sufferers. Many times, these will include things that they wouldn't normally think about. This then leads them to wondering why they would entertain thoughts that are so very unpleasant. As a result, they may believe that this is a sign that they are losing their sanity. The fact is however, that catastrophic thoughts are very common to anxiety disorders sufferers, but it is highly improbable that any of their feared events, will ever occur. While these type thoughts can be troubling and upsetting, they are neither harmful nor dangerous. Click here to see my companion Hub on this subject, titled: "Understanding Anxiety Catastrophic Thinking".

The best way to begin overcoming the fear of catastrophic thoughts, which will in turn also cause them to fade-away and to stop recurring, is to reassure one's self of these facts I have stated, which are backed by reputable anxiety research sources. Thomas A. Richards, Ph.D., Psychologist, for example, states within the pages of his anxiety education resources, that the following catastrophic thoughts may occur with panic attacks:

- fear of losing control

- fear of a stroke that will lead to disability

- fear of dying

- fear of going crazy

- fear of having a heart attack

- fear of passing out

Irrational Fears are Restricting to Quality of Life, but Help is Available

Within Dr. Richard's article regarding the irrational fears experienced by panic attack sufferers, he offers reassurance to those who experience these catastrophic fears, by also stating that these events simply do not occur and that "panic attacks are not in any sense dangerous". If this is true of panic attacks, then this would also be true of the less-intense forms of chronic anxiousness. Search Google, to see Dr. Richard's article titled: "What You Fear the Most Cannot Happen" (use article title as search term). Within this article, the doctor makes it clear that these fears are harmful to the lives of anxiety disorder sufferers, in the sense that they are restricting to them and damaging to their quality of life. Therefore, it is important for anxiety sufferers to seek medical treatment and possible referral by their doctors, to mental health professionals.

Diverting Catastrophic Thoughts with Humor

I, the author of this Hub, have read the testimonials of anxiety sufferers who actually learned to see humor in irrational, fearful thoughts, rather than being terrified of them and this resulted in catastrophic thinking losing its power in their lives. This is of course 'easier said than done', regardless of the replacement thoughts one might entertain to interrupt catastrophic thinking, however, with time and repeated reassuring of one's self, it can be accomplished with very good results. When we think about it, these type thoughts can be humorous and one might even add a little humor to them, as they begin happening! For example, if a person has a fear of losing control, they could add to that thought, the idea of climbing a tree and hanging from a limb upside down by their legs. This might sound like an unusual method for diverting one's thinking, but it can be as effective as any other method, in changing thought-patterns and getting them more under control (thought diversion methods). A final bit of advice I would give however, is that one should not make it a battle or a struggle to change their thoughts, any more than is necessary. Instead, one can almost make a game out of it or see it as an interesting experiment because anxiety seems to thrive on struggle and one should instead attempt to flow with it, rather than to struggle against it.

Defeating Catastrophic Thinking Through CBT

The suggestions I have offered, are an aspect of "Cognitive Behavioral Therapy" (CBT), which is one of the most effective psychiatric treatments for anxiety disorders that exists. Once one gains ground on catastrophic thinking, they will see the struggle aspect of gaining control of their thoughts, fade away and over time, it will automatically be replaced with pleasant, positive thoughts and thinking.

4. Anxiety Sensitization in Thyroid Patients

People who suffer varied degrees and types of anxiety disorders, can experience periods of heightened stress which will in turn, also make them more susceptible to symptoms of chronic anxiousness.

Anxiety is a common symptom listed for thyroid disease conditions. This fact gives good reason for hypothyroid and hyperthyroid patients to learn about anxiety triggers and methods for avoiding or overcoming them. In this article, I will address a phase of basically being "overly-stressed", that people with anxiety problems can reach, that is a precursor to worsened anxiety states. Note: This is not a condition that I have defined but it is addressed commonly by mental health professionals and medical study groups (including the U.S.-NIH) and is also referred to by the names "somatic sensitization" and "cognitive sensitization".

This phase that most anxiety suffers are very familiar with having experienced, as part of their anxiety condition, is best referred to as "Anxiety Sensitization". This is simply a state/phase an anxiety sufferer can reach, when they are experiencing increased stress levels, over prolonged periods of time. This will cause them to reach a heightened state of sensitivity to anxiety feelings. When a person reaches this stage of heightened sensitivity to anxiety, they will experience anxious reactions more easily. Anxiety responses to things will also be more-easily triggered while in this emotional state.

An anxiety sufferer who reaches this state of sensitivity, may become concerned that they have entered a more severe stage of anxiety disorder. These phases, however, are simply temporary increases in anxiety responses and do not indicate a permanent worsening of their disorders. In other words, anxiety sensitization is largely reversible.

When a person is extra tired or extra stressed, they have less resistance to any negative feelings and medical research studies state that there is also less resistance to physical illnesses. Most anxiety sufferers can likely also relate to the fact, that when they are physically weak from an illness, this can also cause anxiety to be triggered more easily in them, because they are in a less-resistant state.

People with anxiety conditions, should observe when they reach this state of becoming sensitized to anxiety, so that they can learn to reverse some of the trends toward getting "stressed out". For example, staying involved in mental studies, such as being on the computer for too long or doing paperwork such as tax returns for extended periods, can result in feeling stressed out (sensitized to anxiety). One should learn to pace their self, instead of taking on too much at a time. It is also a good idea not to take on too many duties at once, in trying to get them all accomplished too quickly. This too, is a stress-producer and we should instead be looking for stress-reducers.

Some ideas for stress-reducing, in addition to the things previously mentioned, would be to take time out to do things that are enjoyable and pleasurable. If one enjoys being outdoors to observe all of the natural beauty and fresh air, they should take time out of their duties and take a nature walk or just sit under a shade tree, with a glass of decaffeinated tea and relax. If exercise is a stress reducer for an anxiety sufferer (as it is for many people), then one should leave their duties behind for a while and get some exercise. This should be done as often as one needs to, to keep stress levels down, as long as they do not exceed their tolerance level for exercise.

Persons with Generalized Anxiety Disorder (GAD), tend to be the type of anxiety sufferers who push themselves too hard and try to get too many things done in unreasonably short periods of time. This many times, is due to their worries about things getting piled up on them if they don't stay ahead of their duties. GAD sufferers also stay busy because it helps them experience some relief from their constant worry and free-floating anxiety feelings. This trend, however, can also end in periods of feeling stressed out, so that there is a vicious cycle of seeking stress relief that instead actually results in causing added stress.

People with GAD and other anxiety conditions, should work on these methods for reducing stress but they should not get overly concerned if they reach these stressed out phases, that cause them to be sensitized to anxiety. The phase will pass and afterward, another opportunity will present itself to again work on eliminating the trends that lead to these phases.

It is also important for anxiety sufferers to remember that if they do reach the point of anxiety sensitization, it will not cause them insanity or death from intense, ongoing periods of anxiety. Adrenaline, the major anxiety producing hormone, can only reach a certain level of placing us on high-alert and then it can go no further (we cannot physically explode from it). The human body is designed, so that it can only metabolize a certain amount of adrenaline at a time. The sensations that come from being overly adrenalized are very unpleasant when they occur "out of context" (when there are no emergencies or dangers present) but they will pass, given time.

One should work on stress-reducing techniques, incorporating exercise, deep-breathing techniques and any other methods that they know will help them avoid those stressed out phases that lead to becoming sensitized to anxiety. With time, it can help them to overcome and conquer "disordered anxiety" in their life.

5. Anxiety with Thyroid Hormone Therapy

If you experience some anxiety symptoms when starting thyroid hormone replacement for hypothyroidism, your case is not unusual, in fact this was my experience when being started on thyroid hormone therapy in year 2003. Patients sometimes experience hyperthyroid type symptoms as their body adjusts to thyroid medication and this can make them feel worse for a while, when anxiety is already there to begin with. Some Doctors help patients through this adjustment period, by giving them an as-needed anti-anxiety medication for use short term use. I say short-term because these as needed anti-anxiety medications can lead to dependency upon them, if taken for more than a few weeks, unless needed for an ongoing anxiety disorder.

Strangely, hypothyroidism can cause anxiety symptoms and some patients seem to experience anxiety when thyroid hormone imbalance is between normal and sub-clinical. The hormone therapy takes a patient to that point between euthyroid (normal hormone levels) and sub-clinical hypothyroidism before it goes on to correct hypothyroidism. This is because as the thyroid medication is brought into one's system, from the outside (orally), their own thyroid begins to shut down any of its own production of thyroid hormone. Some refer to this as "suppression" of the thyroid gland or causing it to "atrophy" (dwindle down). Once a patient gets past that break-even point on thyroid hormone therapy, they can then see improved symptoms as the hypothyroidism is corrected from that point forward. It is a strange but interesting phenomenon and is also why it is referred to as "hormone replacement".

This is just my theory as a well-studied layperson on thyroid disease subjects, but I believe that in-between point of sub-clinical hypothyroidism and that of becoming euthyroid, causes adrenal surges much like people get with hypoglycemia (low blood sugar). The body has an incredible system of sensors, which are the neurotransmitters and the hormones, and it knows how to compensate for hormonal changes. My belief is that when the body senses small downward fluctuations in thyroid hormone, especially when a person is teetering between being euthyroid and sub-clinically hypothyroid, the body tries to compensate for the hormone fluctuation, by releasing more adrenaline, as an alternative source of energy and to keep the body better kick-started. I also believe therefore hypothyroid patients at this point of sub-clinical hypothyroidism, will feel these adrenaline surges upon waking in the mornings. As soon as the patient is awake and ready to start the day, the body senses the need to compensate for inadequate thyroid hormone metabolism, for getting them through the day, and so sends the adrenaline to help out.

This theory of mine comes from corresponding with literally 100s of thyroid patients, in addition to my own experience with this. It also comes from reading several medical research articles that clearly state that anxiety and anxiety disorders, can be related to hypothyroidism, especially with the autoimmune type (Hashimoto's thyroiditis), which is the most common cause in industrialized countries. Some research studies also associate anxiety and panic attacks with sub-clinical hypothyroidism. A patient may need help getting through that in-between stage with the thyroid hormone therapy, by taking an as-needed anti-anxiety medication to help them get there. Also, by self-educating one's self, they lend towards better treatment by becoming a partner with their doctor in working toward getting hypothyroidism treatment optimized, as an individual and unique patient.

6. Characteristics of Bipolar Disorder

I will mention at the start of this article, that I am a layperson and not a medical or mental health professional. There are however many reputable sources that confirm the general facts I include within the information that follows below. Any definitive diagnoses of medical or mental health conditions, must be given by professionals within these fields and this article is offered for general educational purposes only.

I would also mention that emotional disorders are more common in people with thyroid disease, than in the general public. Some published medical research states that thyroid patients develop "lifetime anxiety and depressive disorders", which are rooted in the autoimmune aspect of thyroid diseases. For this reason, those of us with autoimmune hypothyroid and hyperthyroid disorders, should self-educate about these emotional issues. I will now relate some basic information about the manic-depressive condition called "Bipolar Disorder".

With Bipolar Disorder, the name describes exactly what it is, "two opposite poles/extremes". People with it, will become severely depressed, followed by episodes of "mania", meaning periods of exaggerated elation. In fact during these manic episodes, a person can seem to be very energetic and may want to go on a shopping spree for example, or work on a project endlessly and they can actually go without sleep for days or even weeks at a time. They also tend to feel self-exalted at these times, thinking they are very special and greater/stronger than the average person (a type of delusional thinking).

Some bipolar people have "mixed" episodes, in which these depressed and manic spells may alternate more rapidly. The point being, that if you do not experience spells of mania/extreme elation, it is unlikely Bipolar Disorder. Another reason I know this is because I am personally acquainted with people who are bipolar, and it is obvious when a person has this emotional disorder.

I will also relate the fact that when I was in my 20s (now in my 50s), I was suffering for a period of time from both anxiety and depression but these would alternate, in regard to which one was more prominent at certain times. I related this fact to the doctor who attended my medical needs at that time. I also related to him the fact that my extremely stressful job at the time, was the culprit for these emotional problems I was experiencing and that I was losing sleep because of it as well.

Depression alternating with anxiety, IS NOT THE SAME THING. These two commonly co-exist but anxiety is not mania, it is a fear emotion, that also causes chronic worry at times and certainly this would not be considered an elated or exalting feeling. Despite this fact, this doctor diagnosed me with "manic depression" (another name for bipolar) and he prescribed me a powerful anti-psychotic drug, which I ended up only taking for approximately 6 weeks. My discontinuing of the drug was due to my knowing that the doctor's diagnosis was not correct. It also caused me severe side effects and I experienced no benefit from the drug at all.

I would be very cautious in accepting an anti-psychosis drug from a non-specialized doctor who makes a quick-diagnosis of Bipolar Disorder and for a more clear diagnosis, I would see a mental health professional before accepting a prescription drug regimen to treat the condition. Anxiety and depression affect a very large percent of the population, while bipolar only affects an approximate 2.6%.

Depression and anxiety are both strongly connected, and they are also common symptoms of thyroid disease. Bipolar is believed to have a connection to "thyroid autoimmunity" as well but as I describe above, a diagnosis of the condition must also meet the "mania" criteria to be medically recognized as Bipolar Disorder. Prescribed drugs given to people with bipolar, are designed to control the mania aspect of the disorder and to alleviate severe episodes of depression, so that wide swings in emotions to not occur.

Not all people with bipolar hallucinate or become delusional in their thinking -- many do not. Those who do, are not "insane" or "crazy" and being bipolar does not affect one's intelligence negatively. These terms for the psychosis-aspect that can occur in bipolar people and in those with other conditions such as schizophrenia, are unkind and unfair generalizations that should never be directed at people who have mental/emotional conditions that are no fault of their own. Most people with these disorders are productive, contributing citizens to their communities and they can be representatives of every profession in society.

Regular MDs and GPs, in my opinion, should be cautious in diagnosing common anxiety and depression, as psychotic disorders or as Bipolar Disorder and they should test people presenting with symptoms indicating a severe mental/emotional disorder, for possible thyroid disease and other illnesses that can present with symptoms that are similar to them. Doctors should also refer patients to mental health professionals who specialize in bipolar disorder, when in-doubt about a diagnosis of the condition.

7. Hypothyroid Therapy and SSRI Antidepressants

What an amazing subject SSRI antidepressant are, with so many controversies and conflicting opinions out there about them! It is an interesting subject however and one I have searched and researched many times since the year 2003. My searching was also prompted by the fact that I had five doctors in a row try to prescribe SSRI antidepressants to me, during the first 3 years of my own treatment for hypothyroidism. This was because of my experiencing some unresolved symptoms after treatment with thyroid hormone replacement therapy. These doctors felt that hypothyroid treatment drugs are so successful in all patients, that my unresolved symptoms must have been psychosomatic or emotional ones, so they offered me SSRI drugs (I refused them). Once I received the correct dose of thyroid medication however, the symptoms resolved over time, after I was under-treated during the first 3 years.

I believe these antidepressants/anti-anxiety drugs do have a purpose and that there are people who benefit from them tremendously. At times they have probably even prevented suicides. On the other side of the coin however, is the fact that some doctors get into the habit of prescribing them at every turn so-to-speak because they have been so convinced of their widespread compatibility with everyone they might be prescribed to. Some doctors seldom seem to think about those people whom the drugs might not be compatible with, who have adverse reactions to them. Some adverse reactions have also resulted in suicides, but this certainly is not common, although this possibility is now required to be listed on SSRI drug labels.

I feel that these types of possibilities, in addition to other possible severe side effects in patients who are prescribed SSRI antidepressants, shows the need for them to be more thoroughly monitored and educated about the drugs. I feel they should also have a hotline to their doctors when starting these drugs and told to report the first signs of any threatening side effects. Doctors should also be more willing to carefully switch patients to a different type of medication if one causes them adverse side effects. This, rather than telling them that their side effect experiences, are in their heads or just a sign that their emotions were on the verge of getting worse and needing a dose-increase of the SSRI drug.

Some doctors don't inform patients about these things because they are routinely briefed by the pharmaceutical companies who insist that these drugs can be mass-prescribed with very little chance of any adverse effects in anyone who takes them. Again, this does not take away from the fact that the drugs are greatly beneficial to a great many of the people for whom they are prescribed. The reason the FDA has had to step in and require stricter measures regarding the warnings on labels of SSRI drugs, is because severe adverse reactions were happening in some patients taking them. Newly prescribed patients have a right to know about any risks involved in taking them

There are several areas of concern, including those mentioned above, regarding SSRI antidepressants that simply merit more educating of doctors and patients. Patients in need of a trial of one of these drugs may not have the energy to read a long patient print-out that is offered with the medication, so they need their doctors to brief them on all areas of concern in regard to the drugs. One example in this area is the fact that some SSRI drugs and other types of antidepressants require patients who take them to abstain from alcohol and this is another warning some doctors may fail to give them.

Regarding SSRI drugs lowering thyroid hormones in the body, I read about this possibility early on, after I was diagnosed with thyroid disease, regarding the fact that they can indeed do this. I found this information included in medical research articles and not from the opinions of non-medical professional people. In people who take thyroid hormone replacement, this would likely only result in a need to raise their hormone medication dose slightly. In people who aren't hypothyroid however, taking an SSRI long-term, might present the need for them to have their thyroid hormone levels tested every few months, to see if they are a patient whose levels are significantly affected by the SSRI drug. Most patient's, own bodies will adjust their thyroid hormone levels if the drug lowers them over time, but this might not be true in all cases, especially when a person has a hypothyroid disease or is in the process of developing one. Here again, is a need for doctor and patient education about these drugs.

If I were to sum up my opinion on the subject I would simply say that I believe many people are greatly helped by these drugs but I also believe a significant percent of people see adverse reactions and side effects with use of them. I believe that because of this, doctors need to brief patients better about facts regarding possible side effects. SSRI antidepressants are powerful drugs, and, in my opinion, it is extremely important that both doctors and patients become better educated about them.

8. Hypothyroid Therapy for Anxiety-Depression

It is important when a thyroid patient is being treated for hypothyroidism, that they are on as optimal a dose as possible, of "thyroid hormone replacement therapy" (I will abbreviate it as "HRT"). When a patient is placed on a dose of HRT, most will need 1, 2 or 3 dose changes (usually increases) before they reach an adequate/optimal level. When some doctors place a patient on thyroid hormone and the initial staring dose places their thyroid hormone blood-lab levels, anywhere within normal range, some will simply stop there and call it good. They will not afterward, try to "optimize" the patient's HRT (tweaking the dose). This is unfortunate because some patients need more of a "targeted treatment-goal". For example, many patients do not see symptoms such as emotional ones resolve significantly, unless their thyroid hormone dose places their "TSH" level (the most common test used to monitor HRT), at about "1.0". The TSH normal range averages between 0.3 and 4.0. TSH-suppression is the goal because it elevates with thyroid hormone deficiency (hypothyroidism). Some may even need their TSH level at lowest-normal, which is about "0.3 to 0.5", to experience significant symptom relief. A doctor has to be willing to work with a patient, in getting their HRT optimized, by monitoring their symptoms as well as their blood retest lab levels.

Regarding emotional symptoms caused by thyroid disease, anxiety and depression are commonly listed and patients not being treated optimally, may see these symptoms linger. Some treated patients eventually need the addition of an antidepressant and/or an anti-anxiety medication, but some will see their emotional symptoms resolve with thyroid HRT alone. In my case as a hypothyroid patient, once I was treated on the correct dose of thyroid HRT, my emotional symptoms of major depression, resolved within a few weeks. I do have a lifetime anxiety disorder (since childhood), that I must continue to treat but the increased anxiety I experienced during the early onset of my autoimmune thyroid disease, also resolved with treatment (this included frequent panic attacks). Before this however, I was treated by a different doctor who did not optimize my HRT and I struggled with severe anxiety and major depressive symptoms for nearly two years. This doctor kept my TSH between 3.0 and 5.0 and I'm the type of patient who needs a very low TSH (lowest normal, such as "0.3"), in order to maintain symptom control and relief. Not all patients need a lowest-normal TSH to see symptom relief but a good target range to start with, is "1.0". Afterward the level can be tweaked to a slightly lower level, if necessary. Many patients at the "1.0" TSH level, will not need further dose-tweaking.

Some doctors claim that anxiety is not caused by hypothyroidism but that "depression alone" is the emotional symptom of an underactive thyroid. This however is not true. Anxiety is in fact, a common emotional symptom in hypothyroid patients, especially in those who have the autoimmune type called "Hashimoto's thyroiditis (the type I have). Many research studies have concluded this fact. Almost all reputable medical sources list "depression" as a symptom of hypothyroidism and many have added "anxiety" to that list as well. Patients should be pro-active in discussing optimal HRT with their doctors because it is after all, a person's health that is at stake, which affects every aspect of their lives. It is only right that hypothyroid patients be treated, so that they can pursue their livelihood, family needs, enjoyments and all-around quality of life. There are many sensational doctors out there but the ones who don't understand the need to optimally treat hypothyroid patients, should refer their patients to the more specialized doctors, who do believe in "thyroid HRT optimization".

Tweaking thyroid hormones to best possible levels, can be one of the major factors that helps to resolve anxiety and depression problems, in hypothyroid patients.

9. Optimized Thyroid Hormone Therapy Improves Mood

For some treated hypothyroid patients, the emotional-imbalance symptoms of chronic anxiety and depression, can be the ones that are most difficult to see resolved with thyroid hormone replacement therapy. With this being the case, I would like to offer some views regarding the need for optimized hormone therapy, as follows.

It is important that your diagnosed hypothyroid disease be treated optimally because some doctors believe getting TSH (Thyroid Stimulating Hormone levels) and thyroid hormone levels (T4 and T3) anywhere within normal range is adequate treatment with hormone replacement medication. The truth is however, that your better Endocrinologists and Thyroid Specialists have more targeted therapeutic treatment goals. They will for example, have a TSH treatment goal of getting it suppressed down to a "1.0" target range (Normal Range for TSH is usually about "0.3 to 4.0") and as they also consider any remaining hypothyroid symptoms in a patient, they might actually go down to the lowest-normal of from 0.3 to 0.5, to see if a patient has better resolution of symptoms (TSH elevates with hypothyroidism and adding hormone replacement, suppresses it).

Over time, adequate treatment can help a great deal in resolving symptoms such as anxiety and depression. Thyroid medication serves to take over and supply your thyroid hormone needs, while causing your own thyroid gland to be suppressed. You then have more leveled-out thyroid hormones in your body, rather than the erratic changes in levels that a dying thyroid gland produces, when it is trying to make up for a gap in metabolism. This can happen when there is an inadequate dose of hormone replacement, failing to resolve metabolism-needs. When such a struggle is occurring, the fluctuations in thyroid hormones is what gives rise to anxiety symptoms or plummets a patient down into a depressed state or both may occur in an alternating fashion (similar to how Bipolar Disorder works but without the "manic/mania" aspect).

Please go to the Thyroid Health website and read from my article's pages, looking for titles on the "TSH" subject, under the "Medical Testing" category. Also read my articles under the "Anxiety – Depression" category, that will give you some good pointers in regard to treatments for chronic anxiety and/or major depression. Learning not to fear anxiety symptoms, is an aspect of Cognitive Behavioral Therapy (CBT) that I often address, and I have some information in my articles on different aspects of this method. I offer somewhat less about major depression, apart from addressing optimized hypothyroid treatment and anti-depressant medications, simply because it is an emotion that is less active in a person's life (anxiety is pretty much natural for everyday experiences). Depression is also a touchier subject, so-to-speak and it merits caution, due to far more people contemplating suicide from it, as opposed to anxiety disorders -- although this does occur with both.

Some medical sources imply that thyroid hormone replacement therapy, takes only 4 to 6 weeks to do its job but this simply is not true with a large percent of patients, who may need several dose adjustments over several months period, before they reach their optimal treatment level. In the meantime, help with medication for anxiety or depression (anti-anxiety and anti-depressant drugs), is nothing to be ashamed of or afraid of, if you need it while your thyroid treatment is being optimized, which can actually take several months (while the dose is being titrated). Even if you need these types of medications permanently, there is nothing whatsoever wrong with that.

If the antidepressant you're taking for anxiety, is not working as it should (these are prescribed for chronic anxiety) or it is causing unwanted side effects, you might discuss with your doctor, slowly weaning-off of it and also discussing with her an "as-needed" anti-anxiety medication, you can take short-term, rather than the type that must be built-up in your system and maintained. Some patients do fine with the antidepressant types, while others do not. Some doctors seem to believe SSRI drugs and other types of antidepressants work well for everyone, but this simply is not true. I have corresponded with thyroid patients, who simply could not adjust-well to them even after several months of trying to benefit, while many others do very well on them and maintain those benefits.

People are individuals and nothing works the same for everyone and this is a commonsense approach that even doctors should take with prescribed drug treatments.

10. Pros and Cons of the Anxiety Emotion

When you look at lists of symptoms for Graves' disease hyperthyroidism, you will commonly see anxiety and nervousness listed. Many research studies, published on the National Institutes of Health website (PubMed), conclude with the fact that many hypothyroid patients, whose underactive thyroid condition is caused by Hashimoto's thyroiditis, commonly suffer anxiety disorders. Some of these studies state that these are "lifetime anxiety disorders". With this being the case, let's take a look at what this emotion is, how it actually helps us under the right conditions and what it means when it becomes a "disordered" emotion (when it is imbalanced in its manifestations and triggers).

Anxiety is one of the most common emotions we all experience. Without the anxiety mechanism, we might not have the sudden "presence of mind" and the sudden increased ability to react and jump out of the way of an oncoming truck that is barreling down the street, on a direct path to run over us! This mechanism, called the "fight or flight response", that gives us the extra strength and energy, to fight or run, is designed to protect us and so in situations like these (to use an old cliché), "anxiety is our friend".

Anxiety also helps us when we have tasks to perform. People who perform as actors in Broadway plays or have important public speeches to make or a Fireman who has a fire to put out etc..., all depend on the fight or flight response, to enhance their performance and to provide them added inspiration for the task at hand. So again, in cases like these, anxiety is our friend when we can use it for its intended purposes and direct it into positive directions.

Dis-ordered anxiety can cause fears/phobias to develop and to cause ordinary situations to become avoided. One example of anxiety that develops into a "disorder", is when a person becomes fearful of social situations and settings. A certain degree of anxiety is normal in social settings because it lends toward a respectful attitude and helps us put our best foot forward when making friends and acquaintances but when shyness becomes full-blown fear, the anxiety then becomes a disorder.

Another way to look at this, is to say that under normal circumstances, anxiety happens in the "order" it is supposed to. Unfortunately, in some people, the anxiety "fight or flight response", begins to trigger at the inappropriate times, or in a "disordered" fashion. Anything that can be labeled "disordered", can be in the correct "order", just like something that is discolored can become colored.

The way in which anxiety can become a "disordered" thing, is when it does not happen at the appropriate time or is "out of the order" in which it was meant to be. This does not make the anxiety itself an unnatural thing, only the timing becomes unnatural!

11. Psychosis in Thyroid Patients

A few years ago, while moderating on a thyroid disease forum, a close friend of mine posted about being diagnosed by an MD, with "Bipolar Disorder" and they were prescribed an anti-psychotic drug for this. While these type drugs are extremely needful and very helpful to people who do indeed need them for psychotic disorders they are suffering, at the same time I believe any patient in doubt about a diagnosis, should seek confirmation for needing such a drug. Sometimes a second opinion by a qualified mental health professional, is needed because these drugs are powerful and should only be prescribed to patients who have psychotic disorders. It is also a fact published in medical research studies, that newly diagnosed thyroid disease can present similar to psychosis before it improves with treatment.

My friend who asked the question of me, felt that their symptoms simply did not match those listed for the Bipolar Disorder diagnosis they were given. Below was a short article I wrote in corresponding to this fellow thyroid patient regarding bipolar (which sometimes manifests with episodes of psychosis) and their being prescribed drugs for this, despite their concerns that the diagnosis could possibly be incorrect. Some of my article response to this (shown below), came from my own experience in seeing family members diagnosed with psychotic disorders they did not have and from an experience many years ago, when this also happened to me.

Here is that article:

"While I certainly believe these type drugs can be of tremendous value to people who have Bipolar Disorder (the diagnosis your doctor gave you), I also know that for reasons we may never know, there are doctors who are prescribing some of these ant-psychotic drugs to people who do not have the disorders these are designed to treat. I believe the medication your doctor is prescribing for you, is also used to treat epilepsy and migraine headaches.

I know a little about this because I have a nephew and aunt on opposite sides of my family, who were both "diagnosed" with bipolar and schizophrenia and neither of them had either of these disorders.

In the late 1980s, I had a very bad job situation and I developed increased anxiety, due to the stress of it and upon seeing an MD, he diagnosed me with manic depression (similar to bipolar) and prescribed an anti-psychotic drug, which I only took for one month until my Church Pastor made me realize it was a bogus diagnosis and he proved this by showing me a medical resource journal, describing the condition.

My symptoms did not even remotely point to Bipolar Disorder but were typical anxiety symptoms with insomnia, which resolved after a job change, to a less stressful occupation. My advice being in relating this, is to point out that mental health diagnoses can potentially be incorrect if given by doctors who are not specialized in a field. My main suggestion to you, is to see a mental health professional, so that you can place confidence in the diagnosis you have been given or so that you receive a corrected one. You could then move forward with the appropriate medications prescribed, if psychiatric therapy is not offered as an alternative you might rather choose."

12. Psychosomatic Hypothyroid Symptoms?

While researching articles recently, I found some that state to the effect that "patients who do not see their symptoms resolve once optimized on thyroid hormone medication, are simply experiencing added stress and worry from the reality of having the disease". This should not be applied to all treated hypothyroid patients who fail to see adequate symptom-improvement, and these are the type things that have given me passion as a patient advocate, to help bring perspective to this aspect of imbalanced information. It is difficult to stand by silently, when thyroid patients are pegged with these wrong and unfair generalizations, that are simply not true in many cases (weight-gain is an example of a chronic hypothyroid symptom, that is resistant to treatment in some patients).

You would think from some imbalanced descriptions being expressed, that the disease of thyroid autoimmunity, leading to hypothyroidism, is simply a mild condition similar to a cold, that is easily treatable and that seldom ever causes problems once treated. This is why medical research articles being published about the role of "thyroid autoimmunity" in symptoms both physical and emotional and the "Health Related Quality of Life of Thyroid Patients" poles being conducted, are so important in helping to bring balance and perspective to the subject.

Some medical sources and some of the information-pages published by thyroid medication manufacturers, state simply that once a patient with hypothyroidism is on replacement hormone (with most cases being caused by Hashimoto's disease), that they will become completely better and no longer suffer symptoms, after approximately 6-weeks on replacement hormone medication.

While most patients do see significant improvement, many still suffer a degree of symptoms, no matter how optimized their treatments are. This can be attributed to the fact that hormone replacement medications do not cure the underlying autoimmune disease. For this reason, patients should not be patronized, or have it implied to them, that they are hypochondriacs or experiencing psychosomatic symptoms, simply because they do not see complete relief of symptoms from replacement hormone therapy. Patients should instead be instructed on additional treatments that can be self-administered, to gain further symptom improvements. This would include thyroid-improving supplements compatible with their prescribed medications, in addition to improved lifestyle practices.

The doctor I currently receive my own hypothyroid therapy from, also advises me on over-the-counter supplements that can improve my metabolic health, as well as advising me on alterations in my diet and exercise practices, to also improve my metabolism. Thyroid patients should also place effort into researching specialized doctors who can attend them and who understand that the "thyroid autoimmunity" aspect of most hypothyroid cases, requires specialized attention, in addition to the essential, prescribed thyroid hormone replacement therapy.

13. Recognizing Thyroid Patient Anxiety Disorders

Anxiety disorders affect thyroid patients on a more frequent basis than they do the healthy, general population but when does anxiety become a disordered thing? When anxiety is experienced within its proper context, it is not a disordered thing but when it occurs out of context, at inappropriate times and with abnormally high frequency, it becomes a disorder.

Anxiety disorders affect a significant percent of the general population and these include Panic Disorder, Post Traumatic Stress Disorder, Generalized Anxiety Disorder and Social Phobia but when does anxiety become a disordered thing?

How Anxiety Disorders Develop

Anxiety becomes an "Anxiety Disorder", when a person has developed learned behaviors, that cause anxious responses to activate more often than they should, and due to things, that have become triggers for anxiety, that normally should not be. For example: Some people become chronically anxious when they find their selves in social situations. Most people feel a degree of anxiety around people and some may display a high degree of shyness, however, when an abnormally high level of anxiousness occurs when socializing, it then becomes a Social Anxiety Disorder. People with this particular type of anxiety, will experience panicky feelings around groups of people or sometimes even around a single person whom they do not know well.

A Celebrity Who Overcame His Social Phobia

One famous person who overcame his Social Phobia, is entertainer - Donny Osmond. Mr. Osmond noticed his anxiety disorder in childhood, but the condition worsened as he reached adulthood. After experiencing panic attacks while performing on a Broadway stage and when found that he experienced a total dread of having to meet with people, Mr. Osmond sought treatment for his mood problem, via a combination of medications and Cognitive Behavioral Therapy and he has since overcome his Social Phobia

Triggers for anxiety, are also called "phobias", meaning simply "fears" of various things. Some people develop more fears, due to the anxiety reaction itself. This is because the "fight or flight response" itself can be experienced as a "negative" thing by a person (the term for sudden flares of anxiety, including panic attacks). They dread those anxiety feelings when they are in specific situations and they will begin having a negative response to those same experiences/triggers, until they are able to overcome them some point, just as Mr. Osmond overcame his anxiety problems, so that he now enjoys a better quality of life.

Panic Feelings versus Positive Excitement

Other persons exposed to the same situations (such as social settings), might have positive anxiety reactions to them, which we might call "positive excitement". Another example of this would be a person who becomes phobic around snakes and their anxiety response feels very negative to them when seeing a snake and this triggers their phobia (panic feelings). Another person who loves seeing and being around snakes, might become very excited and have just as powerful an adrenaline surge from the fight or flight response, when seeing a snake. However, instead of it causing them to want to run away, it instead makes them want to chase and catch the snake, to take a closer look at it. This is not such a ridiculous example because I, the author, have a nephew, who when he was young, caught many snakes in his childhood and he loved every minute of it, even after being bitten a few times!

Channeling Anxiety into Positive Directions

The point of this look at the term "disorder", as related to anxiety, is so that we can better understand that anxiety can be used positively or negatively in our lives. No one has anxiety mastered to the point that it works for them positively in every situation they experience but it gives each of us a goal in life, for learning to channel anxiety into positive energy as often as we possibly can. We can also work on those phobias, to try and change them into positive experiences, so that the negative feelings begin to fade. This is of course easier said than done but it can be accomplished with practice. One person can experience an adrenaline surge as a very negative experience, such as someone who has a panic reaction to a roller coaster ride, while another person on the same ride, will have just as strong an adrenaline reaction but they will experience it as fun and exciting! This is a basic example of the difference between channeling anxiety into either positive or negative directions.

People with Anxiety Disorders should be encouraged to know that with help through treatments, such as "Cognitive Behavioral Therapy" and other positive treatments, they can learn over time, to change those learned behaviors, so that more anxiety reactions become positive, rather than negative experiences. The first step toward recovery, is to recognize when anxiety has developed into a disorder, so that the need for help can also be recognized.

14. Thyroid Autoimmunity and Chronic Anxiety

Recently while conducting an online search on the subject of the connection of anxiety symptoms to thyroid disease, I found three research articles on the subject, including one titled "Mitral valve prolapse and thyroid abnormalities in patients with panic attacks" (quoted exactly as it appears on the web page). This one is published by the American Psychiatric Association. In the study, they found a strong association between Mitral Valve Prolapse (a common "click heart murmur"), thyroid autoimmunity (presence of TPO antibodies) and Panic Attacks.

Other research articles also associate anxiety symptoms and disorders to "thyroid autoimmunity". While some doctors believe anxiety only happens with hyperthyroid conditions, including the more common Graves' Disease, some medical research states that autoimmune hypothyroidism (Hashimoto's thyroiditis) can also be a cause of chronic anxiety conditions.

Other articles on the subject are available at the PubMed website, published by the U.S.-NIH, regarding anxiety with Hashimoto's disease (use the article titles I am quoting, in a Google search, to locate them quickly). The title of another such article is: "A case control study on psychiatric disorders in Hashimoto disease and euthyroid goiter: not only depressive but also anxiety disorders are associated with thyroid autoimmunity". It is a lengthy title that, also explains the point of the abstract article.

As I have mentioned in other articles I have written, hypothyroid patients have written me by the dozens over the years, complaining of severe anxiety symptoms. Their doctors, however, will sometimes tell them that their thyroid disease is not the cause of their emotional symptoms of chronic anxiety, because they are hypothyroid, rather than being hyperthyroid. This opinion, however, doesn't agree with these research articles, which are looking at the autoantibodies that cause "autoimmune hypothyroidism" specifically (Hashimoto's thyroiditis). These are the "anti-thyroid peroxidase", abbreviated - "Anti-TPO".

A third research article I found during my online browse on the subject of anxiety disorders associated with "thyroid autoimmunity", is titled "The link between thyroid autoimmunity (antithyroid peroxidase autoantibodies) with anxiety and mood disorders in the community: a field of interest for public health in the future". This one is also from the PubMed website. The study states that "thyroid autoimmunity", places patients who are experiencing it, at high risk for mood and anxiety disorders.

I have referenced three medical research articles, that cover the connection of anxiety disorders, to "thyroid autoimmunity" specifically. This makes it very clear that thyroid antibodies, can indeed cause chronic anxiety as part of the symptom manifestations of autoimmune thyroiditis.

15. Thyroid Patients and Panic Attacks

If you have thyroid disease, you may have experienced some co-morbid (related) anxiety along with it. This can especially be true if you have autoimmune thyroid disease, which includes Graves' Disease - hyperthyroidism and Hashimoto's thyroiditis, which can cause Hashitoxicosis (intermittent hyperthyroidism), before it begins causing progressive hypothyroidism.

A very unpleasant type of anxiety reaction is one called "panic attacks" and if you experience them frequently, it is referred to as "Panic Disorder". These are very unpleasant anxiety attacks that cause anxiety symptoms to escalate suddenly. When people experience them, they will often hyperventilate, sweat excessively, experience a racing heart (tachycardia) and extreme fear emotions. If you are a panic attack sufferer, this article is intended to show you that you are far from being alone in experiencing these.

Panic Disorder description and statistics:

"Panic Attacks" are what you might describe as the "climax of anxiety" and they are truly unpleasant, to say the least, as we who have experienced them know! They can occur with just about any other anxiety disorder, including Generalized Anxiety Disorder (GAD) but when the panic attacks themselves are the feature-manifestation, it is referred to as "Panic Disorder" (PD). They can hit extremely hard and a person first experiencing them will commonly believe they are having a heart attack! Many people new to the experience find their selves in hospital emergency rooms, only to be told everything physically checks out normal, once they return to a calmed state. Many new to the panic experience will also believe they are going mad/insane or that another attack will cause them to completely lose control. This is what is known as "catastrophic thinking" but the thoughts are irrational and usually, nothing truly serious takes place as the result of a panic attack.

Approximately 6 million American adults ages 18 and older, or about 2.7 percent of people in this age group each year, have panic disorder, according to the U.S. National Institutes of Mental Health. Panic disorder typically develops in early adulthood (average age of onset is 24), but the age of onset can extend throughout adulthood. About one in three people with panic disorder develops "Agoraphobia", a condition in which an individual becomes afraid of being in any place or situation where escape might be difficult or where help would be unavailable in the event of a panic attack. Agoraphobic people usually only feel safe by staying in their homes and those with severe cases, refuse to venture outdoors or to any other location because of their fear of having additional panic attacks.

Thyroid patients who experience panic attacks, should discuss treatment options for them, with their doctors. In some cases, doctors will refer their patients to mental health professionals, who can administer anti-anxiety therapies. If panic attacks are not frequent-enough to restrict a person's life, a doctor might instead prescribe an anti-anxiety drug therapy.

SECTION SIX

Physical Conditions Caused by Thyroid Disorders

TABLE OF CONTENTS:

1. CFS and Fibromyalgia in Hypothyroid Patients

In year-2006, my blood lab results to monitor my thyroid hormone therapy (for hypothyroidism caused by Hashimoto's thyroiditis), including TSH, T4 and Free T3 (thyroid function tests), were not jiving or correlating with each other. My TSH, at just below 0.2 (the normal range being 0.3 to 5.0), did not match-up with my thyroid hormone levels which were also low.

Usually a low TSH will mean high readings of the thyroid hormone levels or "hyperthyroidism". Patients taking "Armour Thyroid" (the brand of natural T4/T3 thyroid medication that I take) do commonly have a somewhat low T4 level but usually not one that is flagged below normal.

A below normal TSH in hypothyroid patients, usually means over-treatment with thyroid medication but this was not true in my case.

My doctor, an Endocrinologist, raised my 120mg dose of Armour Thyroid, to 150mg. He increased it by 30mg, despite my low TSH. He said that TSH in some patients, does not always accurately reflect some of the other thyroid lab levels. In my case, this was due to my other endocrine glands, including my "pituitary" (the brain-gland that regulates the thyroid), also operating at sub-clinically low levels. My doctor informed me, that this was due to my also having Chronic Fatigue Syndrome (CFS). Many medical sources state that CFS results in a "blunted HPA Axis" (the hypothalamus-pituitary-adrenal axis).

He also informed me, based upon all my test results, including low adrenal hormones, a highly elevated Epstein-Barr Virus count and continually swollen lymph nodes in my throat, that I have co-existing CFS. I had already been told this by a chiropractic doctor, three years earlier. He also added the fact, that thyroid patients sometimes have multi-endocrine gland problems, when everything runs low in addition to the thyroid gland but that this is especially true if a patient also has CFS.

I asked him if CFS was found more commonly in thyroid disease patients and he answered saying "yes, both CFS and Fibromyalgia are more common in thyroid patients" but he added the fact that these syndromes are not often recognized by doctors. This information amazed me because I had seen this Endocrinologist, 4 times previous and I had not asked him up to that point, if he recognized CFS as a real syndrome/illness. He let me know that he certainly did recognized it and that I am only one of several patients he has identified as having CFS.

Several years following my diagnosis of Hashimoto's and CFS, I have improved in many ways. This has been especially true, as my hypothyroidism is treated-well, which reduces and helps to control my CFS symptoms significantly. They do, however, always remain with me to varied degrees and I have learned to tell the difference between CFS symptoms and those of hypothyroidism.

I also asked my doctor if thyroid patients commonly have symptom flares. and he said that any patient with autoimmune thyroid disease will have ups and downs with symptoms, due to antibody and inflammation levels fluctuating. This in-turn causes thyroid hormones to also fluctuate slightly. I believe this is also an aspect that plays a role in the symptom levels experienced by patients with co-morbid CFS and/or Fibromyalgia.

My doctor ordered follow-up blood tests for me after two months on the increased thyroid medication dose, asking for TSH, Free T4 and Free T3 to be tested. My TSH was and is consistently below normal with blood retests, due to my having co-morbid CFS. At the same time, my thyroid hormone levels will be at mid-range and above (up to highest normal), which are the levels most treated hypothyroid patients need to feel well.

I don't often share about my struggles with co-occurring CFS, but I will report that I have done relatively well with it much of the time and I always remain positive about it. I do feel that thyroid patients with ongoing adrenal fatigue could possibly be experiencing a blunted HPA axis and they could be on their way to developing co-morbid CFS, if the adrenal fatigue isn't treated.

If they suspect they have ongoing fatigued adrenals or CFS symptoms, they should ask for their adrenal hormone levels to be tested, preferably by multiple saliva samples over a 24-hour period, to better determine their cortisol rhythm. Cortisol is the "stress hormone" that goes low with different types of adrenal insufficiency (both subclinical and full-blown types).

My doctor did say that treating thyroid disease or any other underlying autoimmune condition is a major factor in helping to control the symptoms of CFS and I know this has been true in my case. I also take adrenal support when needed, that consists of a combination of vitamins, safe herbals and processed bovine adrenal glandular (beef adrenals in pill or capsule doses). These supplements lend toward controlling my symptoms of CFS, by treating the adrenal fatigue which is a major feature of it.

It is an incorrect view for medical sources to state that having thyroid disease, eliminates the possibility of having CFS. This is not true in some cases, in fact autoimmune diseases, including thyroid ones, may be a trigger for causing co-existing CFS and/or Fibromyalgia.

2. Chronic Stress Related Illnesses

Stress is a known trigger for adrenal fatigue and related syndromes, such as Chronic Fatigue Syndrome and Fibromyalgia and can also bring an autoimmune disease to the surface, that is in the body but hasn't fully manifested. Thyroid diseases are some of the more common health disorders that can be triggered by stress, especially Grave's Disease/hyperthyroidism (medical research studies confirm this).

PTSD (Post Traumatic stress Disorder) is also a chronic stress-caused syndrome and is also classified as an anxiety disorder. Studies of patients with PTSD, have shown that they experience a lowering of their adrenal "stress hormones" as a result of developing the condition.

I personally went through an extreme period of chronic stress and my thyroid disease, called "Hashimoto's Thyroiditis", manifested as a result as well as a severe case of adrenal fatigue. I was left untreated for these disorders for several months and as a result I experienced a severe flare in the year 2003, that also triggered the onset of Chronic Fatigue Syndrome.

I initially developed a severe case of hives and a strange viral type illness that left me with the co-occurring CFS. Afterward, the lymph nodes in my neck, remained swollen to this day and I also suffer multiple chemical sensitivities (MCS). These are symptoms characteristic of CFS but that can also occur in people who develop Fibromyalgia.

My belief is that CFS is a syndrome causing an altered HPA Axis (Hypothalamus-Pituitary-Adrenal glands), plus altered immune system function (deficiency). I suggest to people who suspect they have adrenal fatigue, CFS or a chronic illness/disease to have their adrenal hormones and all other hormones (including the sex ones) checked as well because it is my belief that hormonal imbalances over time, can possibly result in CFS and Fibromyalgia type illnesses.

Some who read my articles or my posts on forums, may wonder why I have the passion I do for the "adrenal syndrome" subjects and I would answer that is because of my belief that adrenal fatigue can eventually cause CFS and/or FMS type syndromes, when not diagnosed and treated early when suspected. If a sudden traumatic stressor occurs in a person's life or they go through a period of prolonged chronic stress for whatever reasons, which leaves them with residual symptoms like chronic fatigue or body pain, a visit to their doctor for medical testing, is a good idea.

3. Epstein-Barr Virus a Cause of Hashimoto's?

Medical research has been published regarding the Epstein-Barr Virus (EBV) and its role in causing autoimmune thyroiditis and other autoimmune and neurological diseases. It is also highly associated with different types of cancer. I believe that EBV is the cause of my own Hashimoto's thyroiditis and the resulting hypothyroidism (under-active thyroid), that I began to experience at age 39.

Thyroid disease, especially the autoimmune type runs in families, in fact children of one parent that has thyroid disease, has a 50% chance of also developing the condition during their lifetime. Hossein Gharib, M.D., F.A.C.E, president-elect of the AACE (American Association of Clinical Endocrinologists)and Professor of Medicine at the Mayo Medical School states that "Fifty percent of thyroid disease patients' offspring will inherit the thyroid disease gene."

When I was diagnosed with thyroid hormone imbalance and later diagnosed with Hashimoto's Autoimmune Thyroiditis, I naturally wondered what caused me to have susceptibility to this disease. I knew that thyroid diseases were experienced far more often in women than in men. My mother however does not have thyroid autoimmunity but did develop age-related hypothyroidism, which common in women over the age of 60. I also knew my dad does not have thyroid disease or any other type of autoimmune disease. This is what led me to reflect on any childhood diseases that might have triggered the later life autoimmune thyroid disease I am experiencing because it obviously was not inherited.

I remembered when looking back to my childhood, that I developed a severe case of Mononucleosis when I was about age 10. This is the glandular disease that is caused by EBV and once contracting it -- usually during childhood, the virus remains in your body lifelong. While my siblings (one sister and two brothers), may very well have been exposed to the virus and are likely lifelong carriers now, they did not experience mono as I did. My mono symptoms were the typical ones, including severely swollen lymph glands in my neck and severe fatigue. In fact, I was out of school with the virus, for about six weeks.

My belief is that the virus causing mono in my childhood compromised my immune system and left me vulnerable to developing Hashimoto's thyroiditis which also involves the lymphatic system. Another name for Hashimoto's is "Chronic Lymphocytic Thyroiditis". I feel it is possible, just as the research articles about EBV and autoimmune thyroiditis point out, that EBV causes the immune system over time, to attack tissues in the body that are infiltrated with it, via antibodies it creates to attack it. The immune system is relentless and if it cannot eradicate a virus over time, it may then begin to attack the tissues in the body that contain it (autoimmunity).

When I was rechecked for EBV levels in my blood at age 40 (approximately a year after thyroid disease diagnosis), I had very high titers of the virus still in my system. My result on the blood lab test for EBV antibodies (the antibodies reflect the level of virus cells they are attacking) was "218" with normal values being less that "20". My elevations of the virus, as reflected by this test, were more than 10 times the normal range. While I can never prove with certainty that EBV caused my autoimmune thyroid disease, I will always highly suspect that it is indeed the cause in my case.

4. Epstein-Barr Virus and Chronic Fatigue Syndrome

The EBV (Epstein-Barr Virus), which causes mononucleosis initially in some patients, afterward, remains in a person's body for life. This virus has been long suspected of having a strong connection to CFS (Chronic Fatigue Syndrome). While most people have EBV in their system beginning in childhood (estimates are 80 to 95% of the population), most only have antibody titers to the virus, that are just barely positive, like "5", "10" or "20" points above normal. Others have flares of the virus (reactivation), probably due to a compromised immune system (immunodeficiency) that causes high titers of the virus to increase in their bodies over time.

Many in the medical field are of the opinion that EBV is a background virus like many others in the herpes virus-family, that can flare like cold sores (also a herpes virus that remains in the system). When flares happen, they believe it can cause or at least contribute to symptoms of CFS in some people. In my own case as a CFS patient, my EBV count was "218" when initially tested, with normal range being <20 (below 20), so mine was more than ten times the normal cut off range. It's possible that my doctor ordered a blood test of antibodies to the virus, at a point when mine were flaring, during reactivation of the EBV and when it was highly replicating.

Some Doctors believe the EBV test means nothing, unless being used to test for active mononucleosis but there must be a reason why some patient's EBV counts elevate so highly. Both MDs who treat me for hypothyroidism and CFS, believe that EBV can flare/reactivate in some patients who have the higher titers of the virus in their bodies. Many sources also state that adrenal fatigue is a major feature of this because the adrenal glands are the major moderators of the immune system and they also act as natural anti-inflammatory agents in the body.

While EBV may not be the actual root-cause of CFS, it has been shown to be an indicator of immune dysfunction in studies that have been conducted. In my opinion, it is just one of many factors that can contribute to the symptoms of CFS. The Centers for Disease Control/U.S. Gov. has been publishing studies and diagnostic criteria for CFS, for many years, so it is recognized as a real illness. Many patients with CFS have complete remission of it within two to five years while others have partial but significant improvement, even if it never completely remits. Some may have it for many years but regardless, it does not cause organ damage or decrease lifespan expectancy, according to published medical research. It also does not negatively affect intellect, despite the "brain fog" symptoms it also causes in patients who experience it.

Things that speed recovery for CFS, are treating the associated adrenal fatigue, getting proper sleep and rest, a healthy diet, exercising to tolerance and making sure other diseases a patient might have are also treated (reducing inflammation and added fatigue). Under-treatment of a thyroid disorder for example, can serve as a trigger for continuing CFS flares and may actually be a trigger for the syndrome itself according to some medical sources. Many sources also state that thyroid patients commonly have co-occurring CFS and/or Fibromyalgia (the syndromes have 75% crossover symptoms).

Thyroid patients with CFS should be encouraged to know that symptoms of Chronic Fatigue Syndrome can be controlled, and that complete remission of the illness can potentially occur over time.

5. Fatigue Despite Thyroid Hormone Therapy?

The first thing I always suggest to treated hypothyroid patients who experience low energy and fatigue, which is an important consideration when being treated with thyroid hormone, is making sure it is being as optimized as possible. Some doctors only treat to get the "Thyroid Stimulating Hormone" level suppressed down, to anywhere within the normal range (TSH increases with hypothyroidism) but some hypothyroid patients need a TSH that is very suppressed, in order them to feel better.

The low-normal at most labs for TSH is from about 0.3 to 0.5 and some patients need theirs to be at these lower numbers to see significant symptom relief and a doctor willing to work with them in trials of doses that get them there.

If you haven't received copies of blood labs you've had done to monitor your thyroid hormone therapy, I would ask for your most recent ones, to see where your doctor has placed your TSH level (the "HIPAA" law in the U.S. allows patients copies of labs). If he has kept your TSH level at above 2.0, you may want to discuss a trial of a dose that will suppress the level down to below a 1.0 or even lower-normal.

In non-treated people, the U.S.-NIH suggests that a TSH at 2.0, should be monitored for the possible development of hypothyroidism (in other words 2.0 is a bit too high). Some doctors are overly concerned that getting TSH that low will cause hyperthyroid symptoms however this cannot happen with close monitoring and with a doctor also testing the Free T-3 and Free T-4 levels in patients, for better monitoring of a dose that suppresses their TSH.

Other than this I have mentioned in regard to the TSH level and unrelieved fatigue, I would also suggest that a good multi-vitamin can be beneficial to thyroid patients, especially those with B-12 and the other B vitamins included in them, which can help with energy. The sublingual type (e.g. "Perfect B" or other liquid brands) is good because it absorbs quickly and can be taken twice daily or more, to help energy levels stay up throughout the day.

Some patients also report better symptom-relief and improved energy levels by cutting wheat and dairy from their diet as well (this takes discipline). This is since glutton intolerance (sensitivity to wheat products) is more common in autoimmune hypothyroid patients and dairy products can flare the symptoms of lactose intolerance in them as well.

These are suggestions that may not work for all hypothyroid patients but that can potentially aid thyroid hormone therapy in relieving hypothyroid symptoms, including low energy and fatigue which we would all like to do, best possible.

6. Hashimoto's Disease - A Cause of Chronic Fatigue

While searching for new thyroid disease related information online, I came across a medical research article first published in the "Townsend Letter for Doctors and Patents" and re-printed by Dr. Alan R. Gaby MD. The article reports findings regarding patients with "chronic fatigue", stating that a large percentage of them were found in a medical study, to have the type of lymphocytic thyroiditis that causes hypothyroidism (Hashimoto's thyroiditis). The article is entitled; "Autoimmune thyroiditis as a cause of chronic fatigue".

The interesting aspect of this report is the fact that these patients were not found to have abnormal (outside of normal values) thyroid hormone levels but despite this fact, they were suffering symptoms of hypothyroidism. The autoimmune type of thyroiditis they were suffering from, that was causing the chronic fatigue, was instead diagnosed through a thyroid tissue biopsy called "Fine Needle Aspiration".

What is important about this article, is the fact that hypothyroidism does not have to be present, for autoimmune thyroiditis to cause symptoms. In this case, the research study confirms that the symptom of "chronic fatigue" is one of those that can potentially be experienced, before thyroid hormone levels become abnormal. This study is one of many that confirm the development of symptoms from thyroid autoimmunity in advance of hypothyroidism, detectable through blood testing of the hormone levels. Other medical research articles regarding hypothyroid symptoms caused by the thyroid disease process itself, apart from hormone levels, include patients developing rheumatic and fibromyalgia type symptoms.

In addition to my finding these reports and research for my own articles, these past several years, I have also corresponded with many thyroid disease patients. Many of them also attest to having developed hypothyroid type symptoms from thyroid autoimmunity, in advance of their thyroid hormone levels becoming abnormal. Despite all of this information that is out there and reported by the most reputable medical research entities in existence, there are still doctors who do not believe symptoms can develop in patients with autoimmune thyroid disease, before thyroid hormone levels become abnormal.

In my own diagnosis of autoimmune thyroid disease or "Hashimoto's thyroiditis" -- also referred to as "chronic lymphocytic thyroiditis", I did have abnormal hormone levels (elevated TSH, low T-3 Uptake), in addition to testing positive for thyroid autoantibodies. My hormone levels were not greatly abnormal but the symptoms I was experiencing at the time of diagnosis, including chronic fatigue, were severe in spite my hypothyroidism not being considered "full-blown" (overt) at that point.

Even if there were no research articles stating these facts, it is simply common sense to recognize that the disease process itself has symptom-producing potential. It is after all, autoimmune disease we are talking about and all diseases with autoimmunity as the cause of them, result in inflammation and destruction of tissues within the body that are affected. To think that this type disease process only causes symptoms when it affects hormone levels in the body, takes much of the attention away from the seriousness of that process. Chronic fatigue can be one of the early symptoms of an autoimmune disease process, including that which affects the thyroid gland.

7. Hashimoto's Thyroiditis and Rheumatic Symptoms

Over the past few years, I have corresponded with many thyroid patients with Hashimoto's Disease -- the autoimmune type of hypothyroidism. Patients with the disease complain of many symptoms they experience with this disease that are caused by antibodies attacking the thyroid gland -- eventually causing it to hypofunction.

One of the more common symptoms reported by patients, is mild to moderate "joint and muscle pain". This symptom is also one of those that seems to linger in some patients, months or even years after starting treatment for their hypothyroidism, via hormone replacement medications (T4 and/or T3 therapies).

Some patients experience a worsening of their joint/muscle pain, once beginning a prescribed thyroid hormone drug treatment. This was the experience that occurred in my case, after I began treatment with hormone replacement for Hashimoto's Hypothyroidism. I cannot explain this phenomenon of rheumatic symptom-flares, but I know for a fact that patients do experience it, until their bodies adjust completely to their thyroid medication. As previously mentioned, a percent of patients, continue to struggle with these symptoms, at varied degrees of severity, even after reaching adequate and optimal euthyroid states (normalized thyroid hormones).

What aspect of this disease, results in the concerning symptoms that affect the patient's joints and muscles? There are many contributing factors however, I believe two of the main causes, are inflammation (thyroiditis) and decreased blood circulation, from slowed metabolism.

The inflammation aspect is from the autoimmune process, that causes antibodies to attack the thyroid gland, resulting in high levels of inflammation within it. This inflammation first affects the area of the thyroid gland itself but over time, continuing inflammation can eventually have a systemic affect and travel to other parts of the body.

Autoimmune thyroid disease patients often complain of their joint pain, first manifesting more severely in their shoulders and cervical spine area (upper back). These are the joints that are closest to the diseased thyroid. Over time, these aches can spread to other areas of the body. Some medical research studies state that autoimmune thyroiditis inflammation, can become "systemic" -- meaning it can affect every part of the body to some extent.

Inflammation also tends to lead to stiffness in the joints as well, due to mild swelling and fluid that can build around them. This is caused by the release of "histamines", which are fluids that are sent out by the immune system, acting as agents for overwhelming bacterial and viral intruders and to reduce inflammation.

Most patients see improvement of rheumatic symptoms with thyroid hormone replacement therapy, to correct their hypothyroidism but if relief is minimal, they may need to be blood-tested to detect any co-morbid forms of arthritis and/or connective tissue diseases, including Lupus and Rheumatoid Arthritis.

8. Hypothyroidism and Rheumatoid Arthritis

Patients with autoimmune thyroid disease, should closely monitor their joint symptoms once on treatment for their hypothyroidism. If they find that they have joint symptoms that result in significant swelling or pain that is more than mild to moderate, this could indicate the onset of Rheumatoid Arthritis -- another autoimmune disease, that affects the joints.

There are blood tests, that help diagnose or rule out this disease specifically, the main one being called "Rheumatoid Factor". Two others that are sometimes also used in addition to RA Factor, are the "ESR" (Erythrocyte Sedimentation Rate), which checks for high levels of inflammation and the "ANA" (Anti-Nuclear Antibodies), which tests for autoimmune disease activity. One sign a patient can look for that might indicate Rheumatoid Arthritis is significant swelling and redness in a joint such as a hand, elbow, knee, etc...., that is affected equally on both sides of the body (symmetrical). In other words, with Rheumatoid Arthritis this will manifest in both joints simultaneously, on both sides of the body. Unfortunately, having one autoimmune disease, such as Hashimoto's thyroiditis, places a patient at a higher risk for developing other autoimmune disorders, which is why chronic joint pain should be monitored.

The mild to moderate muscle pain with hypothyroidism which can include cramping and spasms, in my belief is due to a slowing down of all organs in the body, due to lack of thyroid hormone which regulates metabolism. This causes circulation to become less adequate, so that muscles are not nourished by blood and oxygen as they should be. Strangely, some hypothyroid patients experience hypertension (high blood pressure) because the disease causes blood vessels to constrict but at the same time, they may not have proper blood circulation to some of their muscles. This may also occur since heart function is slightly reduced because of the slowed bodily metabolism. This affect also causes symptoms in tendons and ligaments and many hypothyroid patients also complain of "Carpal Tunnel Syndrome" (hand/wrist pain) and "Tarsal Tunnel Syndrome" (pain in the feet).

If a patient has severe, ongoing muscle symptoms, they should seek further medical testing, as previously mentioned regarding joint pain patients, to rule out possible Muscle Disease and Connective Tissue Disorders. Some of the same tests mentioned previously are also used to help diagnose muscle diseases but there are others as well, including one called "Anti-Smooth Muscle Antibodies". There are many Connective Tissue Diseases, including "Lupus" and some patients can experience "Overlap Syndromes", meaning they are experiencing more than one type at the same time.

A well-informed doctor is important when you are being treated for autoimmune hypothyroidism -- one who understands the risks for other autoimmune disease/disorders to develop. A doctor who is highly qualified, can detect when symptoms may indicate something other than thyroid related ones. I personally have visited a few doctors in the past who did not know that hypothyroidism causes joint and muscle pain. Therefore, a truly good, well informed Doctor, is worth her/his weight in gold!

In conclusion I would add that many times, these mild to moderate joint pain symptoms, can be treated with common over-the-counter anti-inflammatory medications. There are also very effective non-prescription, natural supplements that help with joint pain and inflammation, one of these being a combination of "Glucosamine" and "Chondroitin". It is also very important to take your thyroid medication as recommended by your Physician and to let him/her know about other supplements you may wish to take for joint care, in addition to your hormone replacement therapy.

9. Hypothyroidism and Unresolved Arthritic Pain

I was talking to a friend of mine who is being treated for hypothyroidism, who complained that she was not seeing her muscle/joint pain and stiffness resolve with thyroid hormone replacement therapy. She stated that her Doctor had her TSH level (the pituitary hormone that reflects how much thyroid hormone is in the blood) suppressed with the hormone therapy, down to a "3.0". The way TSH or "Thyroid Stimulating Hormone" works in monitoring thyroid hormone replacement therapy is that it is suppressed, meaning it goes lower when more thyroid hormone is in a person's system. I mentioned to her in my response, shown below, that she may not be on a dose of thyroid medication that is enough because some patients need TSH suppressed lower than hers was, in order to see significant symptom relief.

My general response to her:

Yes, hypothyroidism and under-treated hypothyroidism are notorious for causing joint/muscle aches and stiffness. This was a major symptom for me, before I was well treated, and it was the symptom that best resolved for me and that remained improved for several years after my hormone replacement was better optimized. While I do suffer from arthritic/rheumatic symptoms now, this is due to my developing other conditions since that time.

There are Doctors who will treat hypothyroid patients with thyroid hormone replacement, by only getting their TSH down to around 3.0 or 4.0 but according to medical sources, some patients do not feel well or see some symptoms resolve well, unless their TSH is suppressed down to about 1.0 or even slightly lower. Doctors, who avoid suppressing TSH down this low, are concerned about inducing a hyper-toxic state or hyperthyroidism, caused by too much thyroid hormone medication. The fact is however, that lowest-normal is approximately from 0.3 to 0.5, so getting TSH down to 1.0 or even between 0.5 and 1.0 doesn't place a patient at risk for medication-induced thyrotoxicity. In addition to this fact, the fear of inducing hyperthyroidism, gives way to keeping a patient in a state of unresolved symptoms and one must wonder why ongoing hypothyroidism would not also be looked at as serious for the patient as well.

The new TSH guidelines as revised by the American Association of Clinical Endocrinologists, in 2002, is "0.3 to 3.0", which places 3.0 at highest normal. This would now be considered borderline hypothyroidism. The National Institutes of Health, on the MedLinePlus website, states on their page titled " MedlinePlus Medical Encyclopedia: TSH", that "If you are being treated for a thyroid disorder, your TSH level should be between 0.5 and 2.0 mIU/L". A TSH reading such as 1.0 fits within that therapeutic range for treatment of hypothyroidism.

Strangely, there are Doctors who can see these sources, which are the most reputable in the world and they will still disagree with them. In my opinion, when you have a Doctor not willing to work with you in optimizing your thyroid hormone therapy, using these suggested guidelines, it is time to find one who is willing to better treat your hypothyroidism.

10. My Thyroid Disease CFS and Adrenal Fatigue Story

My ongoing battle with adrenal fatigue began to manifest even before I experienced the obvious onset of Hashimoto's/Hypothyroidism in early 2003. I noticed months before diagnosis, that my tolerance for stress and my recuperative abilities, to spring back from hard physical activity, illnesses, excessive stressors etc.., was slowly diminishing. When my hypothyroid disease kicked in, the adrenal fatigue hit a peak of severity and the combination of the two really threw me for a loop.

The first Doctors I visited, didn't investigate to find the thyroid disease and I was not being treated for it, so in the meantime I had to push myself incredibly hard just to keep going. I also had an extremely stressful job in property management at that time.

Finally at one point, the adrenal fatigue turned into severe "adrenal exhaustion" and I experienced a strange viral type illness that left me with severe hives (these resolved) and swollen neck lymph-nodes that have remained swollen to this day. This is also when my chemical sensitivities became much worse to caffeine chocolate, alcohol and stimulants of any kind. In other words, I had developed increased multiple chemical sensitivities (MCS).

I finally demanded blood tests and as a result, I was treated for diagnosed hypothyroidism, but the adrenal fatigue remained, recurring in flares of symptoms. Over time, I learned the difference between the symptoms of adrenal fatigue/exhaustion and thyroid symptoms. With adrenal exhaustion, I experience severe post-exertion malaise and it can take a couple of days sometimes to recuperate from hard physical activity.

I have since been treated for these health disorders and have seen significant improvement in them. I do still experience flares of symptoms, if I venture outside of a diet restricting stimulants or if I do not keep my stress levels under control.

It is my belief that Chronic Fatigue Syndrome (CFS) has as a feature of it, a type of adrenal exhaustion (one major aspect) and that a milder adrenal fatigue can be a forerunner to it in some cases. One of the most well-established features of CFS that you find in medical research (also fibromyalgia), is "low cortisol levels" and I do not believe this is a coincidence but something that makes sense because the main purposes of cortisol is regulating stress and controlling inflammatory responses in the body. Two of the doctors I have been treated by since 2003, also diagnosed me with co-morbid CFS.

The adrenals when low functioning, cause more allergy, viral and illness responses to occur, due to the role of the glands in immune system function. Cortisol is also our body's natural anti-inflammatory and so low levels give rise to joint and muscle pain, and other inflammatory reactions in the body. All of these factors combined, contribute to the symptoms of adrenal fatigue and CFS and can add to the symptom-struggles of hypothyroid patients who have these co-morbid conditions.

11. Thyroid Autoimmunity and Hives-Rash

In recent years, medical research has found a strong connection between thyroid autoimmunity and skin hives or what is medically known as "chronic uticaria". Some of the studies specifically state that "Hashimoto's thyroiditis" can be a cause of recurrent hives. Yet even more medical research studies have shown that children with chronic hives or uticaria should be screened for autoimmune thyroid disease by blood testing their thyroid hormone levels and by also testing them for "thyroid antibodies".

The two types of thyroid antibodies (also called autoantibodies), that are most common in causing autoimmune thyroid disease are the "anti-thyroid peroxidase" antibodies (Anti-TPO) and the "anti-thyroglobulin" antibodies (Anti-TG). If either or both are found to be positive in patients with chronic hives, this could be an explanation for their cause.

When I was personally diagnosed with hypothyroidism in early 2003, one of the symptoms I experienced that told me something unusual was occurring in my body, was a severe case of hives. I experienced these, just before worsening symptoms of hypothyroidism, also began to occur. I had never experienced uticaria before this from either allergies or from stress and I felt they were a strong indication that something serious was going on with my immune system. It was in fact thyroid autoimmunity that was flaring in my system and the hives were a result of this chronic immune response that was destroying my thyroid gland and causing me to also experience progressive hypothyroidism (under-active thyroid).

The doctor I visited when the hives were flaring up, felt that I was experiencing a food allergy, but this had never happened before. I instead thought it was an allergy to a plant of some type because I had been doing a lot of landscape work at that time, while managing some property. The job I had at the time was also very stressful and so I also considered the severe stress as a possibility for the hives outbreak. The fact is however that I was experiencing the onset of hypothyroidism, from Hashimoto's thyroiditis. I feel the disease hit a level of severity, with stress as a possible contributing factor, that caused my body to release histamine (fluid produced by the immune system to fight allergens) which surfaced on my skin, as a severe case of uticaria.

The PubMed medical research website, provided by the National Institutes of Health and the National Library of Medicine, published an article titled: "Association between chronic urticaria and thyroid autoimmunity: a prospective study involving 99 patients." The article states the following conclusion: "This study shows a significant association between chronic urticaria and thyroid autoimmunity, and that tests to detect thyroid autoantibodies are relevant in patients with chronic urticaria, whereas extensive laboratory tests are not." (Quotes in print are allowed for public education)

When chronic hives (uticaria) is experienced and it is an unusual occurrence not easily explained by an allergen or another obvious cause, a patient should see their doctor and request thyroid antibodies and thyroid function tests to be ordered. These tests can rule out thyroid autoimmunity or help to confirm it as being the cause of this condition.

12. Thyroid Disease and Diminished Libido

There are many concerning symptoms that can occur with thyroid disease but one of the more concerning ones is "loss of libido" -- meaning a decreased sex drive. One reason this symptom can be so concerning is because of the possible strain it can place on the marriage of a thyroid patient. I know this concern to be a very real one because I have corresponded with both male and female patients with this problem on public thyroid forums, over the past several years. It is of such great concern to some of them, that it can cause them depression symptoms as well.

Thyroid patients who usually have more of a problem with loss of libido are those with hypothyroidism. Those with hyperthyroidism can also experience this symptom but they may also experience episodes of increased sex drive, due to the sped-up metabolism hyperthyroidism can causes. With hypothyroidism, the metabolism is slowed down, which means the reproductive organs are slowed down as well. The adrenal glands that produce cortisol and DHEA hormones, convert them into sex hormones (estrogen and testosterone). However, this process is slowed down and both men and women can see decreased levels of both adrenal and sex hormones.

The good news is that when thyroid hormone imbalances of either the hypothyroid or hyperthyroid types are corrected, the result is a normalizing of all bodily hormones and functions, including a somewhat restored sex drive (in relation to a person's age). Many thyroid patients report that they regain a certain degree of their libido back although many reports say that it is not back to 100% of what it was before the onset of thyroid disease. To regain a significant percent of virility however is far better than to remain in an almost void state of libido.

There are also prescription drugs that can help men in this area and the reason this is slightly more of a need for men, is due to the fact that they rely upon a bodily function, that if not operating properly, prevents intimacy with their partner from taking place. This fact is also the reason lack of libido can seriously affect some men psychologically because they feel lack of ability to perform sexually, brings into question their masculinity and ability to satisfy their partner. This then leads them to worry about their marriage in general. Certainly, this is also a concern for women who also have problems with being responsive to their husbands, due to decreased libido. In addition to drugs that can help, there are also hormone therapies that can be administered by a treating Doctor, if sex hormones are found to be insufficient and in need of additional hormone therapies to correct them.

Thyroid hormone therapy must sometimes be given several months of time, to help in areas such as libido because it can take this much time to see all bodily organs regain a significant degree of their pre-disease functions. If libido is not adequately restored with thyroid hormone replacement, patients should remember that their doctors may be able to suggest additional drug or hormone therapies as described above, that can help in this area.

13. Thyroid Disease and Hair Loss

A symptom that is listed for both hypothyroid and hyperthyroid conditions is "hair loss". Some patients, especially those with hyperthyroidism, may see rapid hair loss with their thyroid disorder. Other patients only see mild to moderate hair loss, such as finding more hair in the sink after washing it. Hypothyroid patients will find that their hair becomes dry and brittle and will also break off rather than just falling out.

Some thyroid patients being treated for hypothyroidism will report that they experience hair loss, more so with a thyroid hormone replacement medication. The thinning hair they experienced prior to starting hormone therapy was mild to moderate or in some cases almost unnoticeable but once starting thyroid medication, they see a rapid increase in losing hair. I have seen this attested to, more often in patients taking synthetic forms of thyroid hormone medications, while other patients are not affected with hair loss by synthetic or the natural types of thyroid hormone medications (animal derived).

In my case, as a hypothyroid patient, I experienced mild hair loss when I began experiencing symptoms of hypothyroidism from Hashimoto's thyroiditis (an autoimmune disease and the most common cause). I would find a half-dozen or so hairs in my sink after hair-washing and possibly a few hairs on my pillow upon waking in the mornings, but I didn't see moderate or severe hair loss at that time.

At one point during my thyroid hormone therapy however, I was switched from Armour brand, natural thyroid medication to Thyrolar, a synthetic combination T4/T3 medication. After about two weeks on Thyrolar, my hair began to fall out in moderate amounts. I actually was only switched from Armour, to see if mild intermittent hives I was experiencing were due to it causing me an allergy but after over a month on Thyrolar, the mild hives continued and so they were attributed to my thyroid autoimmunity and not caused by the type thyroid medication I was taking. With this being the case, I asked to be switched back to Armour and the hair loss stopped.

Patients are individuals and none of the scenarios I described are true of everyone. It is also true that most patients taking a type of thyroid medication that does cause them hair loss will see this side effect resolve, given additional adjustment-time on their thyroid hormone therapy. One importance in the hair loss symptom in people, who are not on thyroid hormone therapy, is recognizing the fact that it can be an indication of thyroid hormone imbalance, especially in people who are experiencing other symptoms that may indicate a change in their thyroid function.

14. Thyroid Disease and Mitral Valve Prolapse

In other articles I have written on the "Mitral Valve Prolapse" subject, I make mention of the association between this common heart "click murmur" and autoimmune thyroid disease. I have since, expanded my search and research on this connection and have found no less than five highly reputable research groups reporting on this association.

What does this mean for thyroid patients? The medical reports themselves state that this fact demonstrates the importance for thyroid patients in being tested for this heart murmur. Some of the research also states the possibility that MVP also has an autoimmune component to it or that it may be an autoimmune disease itself. While many patients with this heart abnormality do not experience symptoms, those who do are termed as having "Mitral Valve Prolapse Syndrome" (MVPS), the syndrome aspect, being a reference to the array of symptoms it can cause.

The symptoms of MVPS include:

* Dizziness upon first standing

* Wide swings in blood pressure

* Fatigue and exercise intolerance

* Shortness of breath, especially upon lying flat

* Spells of racing heart, skipped beats and flutters

* Anxiety and depression

Some of the symptoms related to this heart murmur, are a result of what is called "dysautonomia", meaning the involuntary nervous system (INS) becomes slightly imbalanced, causing a usually mild failure in blood pressure regulation and an imbalance in other involuntary bodily functions (each under the influence of the INS).

It is very likely that people who already have MVP but who also experience the onset of autoimmune thyroid disease (Graves' disease or Hashimoto's thyroiditis), may see the MVP/MVPS worsen in symptom manifestations. It is also possible that thyroid autoimmunity itself, serves as a trigger for causing MVPS. This must be considered because medical studies have shown the condition to be very common in thyroid disease patients, as opposed to control groups (non-thyroid disease participants in their research studies).

Professor Bell, director of the endocrine clinic at the University of Alabama School of Medicine in Birmingham, AL has reported finding MVP present in 41% of patients with Hashimoto's thyroiditis and in 41% of Graves' Disease patients who were studied. (as reported by WebMD)

Professor M.E. Evangelopoulou and colleagues from Alexandra Hospital at Athens University School of Medicine reported an average of 1 in 4 patients with Graves' and Hashimoto's, as having comorbid (associated) MVP. None of the healthy people in the control group without thyroid disease were found to have MVP. (title of the study: "Heart Valve Defect Common in Patients with Thyroid Disease")

The American Journal of Psychiatry published a study in 1987, stating that there is a strongly confirmed association between panic attacks, mitral valve prolapses, and autoimmune thyroid disorders. (title of the study: "Mitral valve prolapse and thyroid abnormalities in patients with panic attacks")

Several studies are also published on the National Institutes of Health-National Library of Medicine medical research website. One of the studies states that "the prevalence of mitral valve prolapse is significantly increased in patients with autoimmune disorders of the thyroid gland, when compared to normal and non-autoimmune conditions" (title: "Prevalence of mitral valve prolapse in chronic lymphocytic thyroiditis and nongoitrous hypothyroidism." - Quotes allowed for public information sources)

Another important aspect to this subject is the fact that thyroid patients, who have MVP/MVPS, may in fact confuse the symptoms of the heart murmur with unresolved thyroid disease symptoms being treated. Some medical sources also state that people with MVPS may sometimes be diagnosed as having Chronic Fatigue Syndrome/"CFS" (due to ongoing fatigue the syndrome can cause). Another connection regarding CFS to the click murmur, is the fact that people suffering the condition often have dysautonomia which can also occur with MVPS.

I see in this subject of MVP being strongly associated with autoimmune thyroid disease, the importance in recognizing how commonly comorbid (associated) some conditions are and the importance in considering these connections when treated thyroid patients are not experiencing the expected symptom relief from treatments. Doctors should recognize the need in testing for MVPS via echocardiograms, in patients whose unresolved symptoms may match those for Mitral Valve Prolapse Syndrome/Dysautonomia.

15. Thyroid Disease and Orthostatic Hypotension

Have you ever felt dizzy for a few seconds after standing up from your chair? If so, you may have experienced an episode of a common condition called "Orthostatic Hypotension".

Orthostatic Hypotension (OH) is also referred to as Orthostatic Intolerance and in its simplest form, it simply means that you get dizzy upon standing up from a seated (supine) position. This phenomenon is in the "dysautonomia" category, which is a form of involuntary nervous system dysfunction. When this part of our nervous system has mild to severe imbalances in it, due to disease processes within the body, things that normally function properly in our bodies, such as blood pressure and heart rate, are slightly off-balance. In the case of Orthostatic Hypotension, blood pressure does not rise as it is normally supposed to with positional changes of the body, going from seated/lying down to standing up, but instead it drops slightly, resulting in the symptoms of OH.

The symptoms of OH include dizziness that lasts a few seconds, a feeling like you are about to black out, a pressure sensation in the neck, head and chest area, temporary rapid heart rate (tachycardia) and a temporary change in vision. These symptoms are a result of the drop in blood pressure and they subside once the body adjusts to the change in body position and blood pressure returns to normal.

Some people have more severe forms of OH and their blood pressure remains dis-regulated even after their body should normally have had time to adjust to positional changes (this steady imbalance is sometimes termed "Orthostatic Intolerance"). The more severe type of dysautonomia, is also referred to as Postural Orthostatic Tachycardia Syndrome (POTS), which causes an array of symptoms throughout the body. People with this type of dysautonomia are usually medically treated for their condition while milder forms of orthostatic hypotension do not usually require treatment.

Diseases and conditions that can cause Orthostatic Hypotension are usually endocrine disorders and syndromes that influence adrenal gland function, such as Fibromyalgia, Post Traumatic Stress Disorder and

Chronic Fatigue Syndrome. A common "click heart murmur", called Mitral Valve Prolapse can also cause dysautonomia symptoms, including OH and when it does, it is referred to as "Mitral Valve Prolapse Syndrome".

Other health disorders such as anemia, hypovolemia (low blood volume) and dehydration can cause OH and certain types of medications can potentially cause it as well, including drugs for hypertension and certain types of antidepressants. Many thyroid patients also complain of suffering symptoms of Orthostatic Hypotension, especially those who have Grave's Disease but patients with hypothyroidism can also experience it. Many people who experience OH, have no known distinguishable cause for it (idiopathic).

The treatment for OH is usually simple lifestyle changes when it is mild to moderate, including exercise and eating healthy, making sure there is ample salt in the diet (if hypertension is not present) and drinking plenty of water which helps to keep low blood pressure episodes from occurring (hypotension). When drug therapy for OH is used, it may include "Fludrocortisone" (Florinef), which is a mineral-corticosteroid used to help regulate blood pressure, "Midodrine" (alpha-1 adrenergic agonist), "Methylphenidate" (amphetamine) and "Ephedrine" (adrenaline stimulant). These drug treatments are not recommended or prescribed however, when lifestyle and diet changes are able to control the symptoms of OH.

16. Thyroid Disease and Peripheral Neuropathy

Many thyroid patients complain of neurological type symptoms and many struggles with these even though they are well treated to correct their thyroid hormone imbalance. Other endocrine diseases, such as diabetes can cause symptoms of neuropathy, as well as neurological disorders that originate from within the brain. "Peripheral Neuropathy" is a term meaning a patient suffers from nerve-related symptoms in their body, that extend out to the extremities. It can affect nerves that travel to any parts of the body, from the Peripheral Nervous System, so that there is a systemic type effect -- meaning there are many areas of the body affected (body wide, such as with Fibromyalgia).

The symptoms of neuropathies can include tingling and numbness sensations in the body, but the extremities are more-commonly affected (hands and feet). It can also include burning sensations and stabbing type pains. Muscle twitches and tremor in the muscles can also be a common symptom of peripheral neuropathy. This particular symptom of tremors affects many thyroid patients with Grave's Disease (autoimmune hyperthyroidism) but it can also manifest in those with Hashimoto's thyroiditis (autoimmune hypothyroidism).

Some patients with neuropathy type symptoms may also complain of symptoms such as "tinnitus" -- meaning ringing, roaring or clicking sounds in their ears. Some may also experience a degree of hearing loss and dizziness, caused by the imbalanced nerve signals reaching the inner ears.

In the year 2007, I personally had a Brain MRI performed, due to experiencing the variety of symptoms I describe above. My test result came back negative for signs of neurological disease, which this confirmed to me and my doctor, that my peripheral neuropathy was caused by autoimmune thyroid disease (Hashimoto's - Hypothyroidism).

Some medical sources state that neurological symptoms are rare in thyroid disease patients with hypothyroidism however this is not what I've been hearing from 100s of patients over the years since 2003, who attest to experiencing neuropathies, despite being well-treated with thyroid hormone replacement therapy. My belief is that these symptoms may originate from thyroid antibody levels (autoimmunity) and not from thyroid hormone imbalance.

There is a severe condition that can occur in patients with autoimmune hypothyroidism, called "Hashimoto's Encephalitis", which causes severe neurological symptoms and is caused by thyroid antibodies, however, it is a very rare disorder. It can present with epileptic seizures, amnesia, psychosis and even coma or death, if not treated very soon after being diagnosed. I feel there are lesser degrees of peripheral neuropathy illnesses, related to thyroid antibodies and that it is only common sense to recognize that they can cause neuropathies that are milder than those of Hashimoto's Encephalitis.

If you are a thyroid patient experiencing peripheral neuropathy symptoms, discuss with your doctor any testing you might need, to rule out causes other than your treated thyroid disease.

17. Thyroid Hormone Therapy and Heart Palpitations

Heart skip palpitations are also referred to as "Premature Ventricular Contractions" ("PVCs" - which are actually premature/extra heartbeats, that feel like skipped ones). In hypothyroid patients, these can sometimes occur when they are taking thyroid hormones, to replace those that are low in the body. With hormones apparently playing a factor in these sometimes scary palpitations, one should not only avoid the other known triggers for PVCs, such as extra stressors, sleep deprivation and consuming too many stimulants (i.e. caffeinated coffee/tea, alcoholic beverages and manufactured sugars), but one should also attempt to keep their hormones properly balanced as best possible. This would include thyroid hormones that are being taken as replacement therapy for hypothyroidism.

In order to accomplish this, hypothyroid patients should report any symptom-changes in their treated underactive thyroid conditions, to their doctors, in case a new blood test needs ordered sooner than scheduled to determine if a dose-change in the therapy is needed. The daily dose prescribed should be taken faithfully, usually first thing in the morning on an empty stomach (at least 30 minutes before eating), with plenty of water to help it absorb into the system. Any supplements or foods with high calcium or any iron in them, should not be consumed until 6 hours after a thyroid dose is ingested (these can hinder its absorption).

While some patients develop hypothyroidism as the direct result of a disease within their glands, others develop it as the expected after-effect of treatments for hyperthyroidism (e.g. following thyroidectomies or RAI ablations). Either way, thyroid hormone replacement therapy is the required life-long treatment, for which there is no alternative.

Patients whose hypothyroid therapies are well-regulated as reflected by optimal normal-values blood test results of their TSH, T3 and T4 levels, only need retested, every 4 to 6 months once a euthyroid state is achieved (normalized metabolism). Testing may need to be repeated sooner however, if symptoms manifest between blood retests that are scheduled this far ahead, and this should include the onset of heart palpitations of any type. Not only can "ectopic heartbeats" signal an abnormal change in thyroid hormone levels (yet another name for PVCs) but other types of palpitations can as well, including tachycardia (a fast heart rate, possibly indicating over-treatment with thyroid hormone) and "bradycardia" (a slowed heart rate, possibly indicating under-treatment). NOTE: Bradycardia is defined as a resting heart rate of below 60 beats per minute, while tachycardia means the heart rate is 100 beats or more at rest.

If additional medical treatment is needed for heart palpitations, this will usually be a beta-blocker medication (a drug usually prescribed for hypertension that partially blocks the effects of adrenaline in the body) and lifestyle changes to modify diet and exercise practices. There are different classes of "anti-arrhythmic drugs" available as well, however, doctors usually prescribe these for the more serious types of heart arrhythmias rather than for benign ectopic beats which are usually not considered a risk-factor for anything potentially serious in otherwise heart-healthy individuals.

SECTION SEVEN

Adrenal Fatigue in Thyroid Disorders

TABLE OF CONTENTS:

1. Adrenal Fatigue - The Stress Syndrome

There is a commonly experienced health problem that is beginning to be recognized by more Doctors, called "Adrenal Fatigue". It is also known by the names "Adrenal Exhaustion" and "Low Adrenal Reserve".

This condition, which causes characteristic symptoms (syndrome), has become increasingly common over the past several decades. The main symptoms caused by Adrenal Fatigue, include:

* fatigue

* low tolerance for stress

* joint aches

* low tolerance for exercise

* irritability, anxiety

* depression

* low resistance to allergies and sicknesses

* sugar & salt cravings, and overuse of caffeine

The reason for the craving of these substances last mentioned, is due to the need to supply energy from other sources, due to the person's adrenal glands having the diminished ability to do so.

This brings us to the understanding of what this syndrome is. It is a syndrome of the adrenals, that have become exhausted, due to prolonged, chronic stress that has been placed upon them. The adrenal glands, which are two small glands, one sitting on each of our two kidneys, are designed to give the human body, the ability to handle and spring back from stress. They do this by means of releasing hormones, that circulate throughout the body, giving it coping abilities and energies to deal with stressors. These stressors are anything, mental or physical that place a demand of any kind on our bodies. This means stressors can be positive or negative but either type will place demands upon the adrenal glands.

The most important hormone released by the adrenals that helps us deal with stress, is the one called "cortisol" or "cortical". It, like the hormone adrenaline, is also a "fight or flight" hormone. The difference between them being that adrenaline is the hormone to help us with immediate need for increased bodily functions to deal with tasks at hand needing performed. Cortical on the other hand, is the long-term fight or flight hormone, that gives us a steady ability to handle all our everyday stressors.

With today's fast-paced society and the increased demands for stress-coping, it is very easy for people to overuse their adrenal reserves, giving them inadequate rest and time, to rebuild their stress hormone resources. By not getting enough sleep after overwork, plus adding other bodily stressors, such as bad diet and overuse of caffeine, refined sugar and other stimulants (including tobacco), the adrenals eventually begin to run down. Once a person reaches this state, they begin to experience the concerning symptoms that result from this very real "stress syndrome".

2. Adrenal Fatigue and Thyroid Patients

Experiencing the onset of a thyroid disease, is already a stressful thing. When adding more stress to the mind and body, Adrenal Fatigue can also begin to manifest.

Many patients with thyroid disease also have some co-existing adrenal fatigue, in fact some medical statistics show that there is some degree of adrenal hypofunction, in up to 10% of all thyroid patients. The term "adrenal fatigue", simply refers to a sub-clinical lowering of adrenal hormones in the body (within normal values but at the lower end) but not an actual clinical lowering of them (below normal values – overt deficiency), which would be identified as "adrenal insufficiency". The two hormones that drop to near sub-normal levels with adrenal fatigue, are "cortisol" -- the stress-regulating hormone and "DHEA" -- the full name for this one being "Dehydroepiandrosterone", which converts into the needed sex hormones in both males and females.

How Does Adrenal Fatigue Occur?

Add to thyroid disease or other chronic illnesses, something such as a traumatic or very stressful event and one can really begin to suffer from adrenal fatigue. Cortisol circadian rhythms become off with this condition and therefore sleep patterns become disrupted. Cortisol and DHEA will have their peaks, at the wrong times, such as at sleep-time and the normal rhythmic drop in these hormones will also happen at the wrong times, such as during the day when one is in the most need for peak energy (such as during daytime work hours). Adrenal fatigue that continues for prolonged periods (chronic), can then become "adrenal exhaustion" and this is the point at which a person may no longer experience those needed peak levels at all.

Being a thyroid disease patient myself, I have experienced adrenal fatigue for several years, as a feature of Chronic Fatigue Syndrome and I have also experienced adrenal exhaustion. Mine turned into adrenal exhaustion, after experiencing the onset of Hashimoto's/hypothyroidism (autoimmune thyroiditis) and at approximately the same time-period, I was going through a terribly stressful period with a properties management job I held at the time.

How I Treat My Adrenal Fatigue

Mine did not improve when I first began thyroid hormone replacement therapy, but it worsened for a time. This is a phenomenon that thyroid hormone manufacturers warn about possibility occurring, when untreated adrenal hypofunction is present at the time hypothyroid drug therapies are started. After several months on the correct thyroid hormone dose, I eventually saw some improvement in hypothyroid and adrenal fatigue symptoms. At times of extra stress and extended periods of hard physical activity, however, I have learned to take some adrenal support supplements, that I discovered when researching about adrenal fatigue and these have helped me in this area. These include multi "B" vitamins, especially B-12, in sublingual form (liquid), B-5, B-5, C, magnesium, selenium, zinc, DHEA 25mg (over-the-counter adrenal hormone) and sometimes but less-often, I have taken an Adrenal Cortex Extract (beef adrenal glandular, processed into pill form).

These help me a great deal, but I don't take the ones containing actual adrenal hormone (cortisol - found in some glandular supplements), as a permanent regimen. As safe as they are supposed to be at the recommended doses, it likely would not be harmful for me to do so, if I felt it was necessary but I always err on the side of caution and only take them "as-needed".

I considered taking a cortisol hormone drug called "Cortef" at one point (natural adrenal steroid) and I was seeing a doctor at the time, who was willing to treat me with the medication but I was a little wary of steroids and I declined the treatment. I have since however, read many reputable medical resources stating that Cortef is safe at physiological doses (25mg and less), to supplement a person's low cortisol levels from adrenal exhaustion. It can however, cause "adrenal suppression", if administered in full replacement doses (above 25mg, which may vary among individual patients) and if used for extended periods of time. In my opinion, adrenal support supplements that boost the adrenal glands into producing their own cortisol, are safer and usually all that is needed for most cases of adrenal fatigue.

How Does a Patient Know if They Have Adrenal Fatigue?

Single blood adrenal hormone levels can be helpful, but they are like a "snapshot reading" and since cortisol levels go up when you are stressed (such as at a blood draw), this can affect the snapshot blood level. Therefore "saliva testing" is recommended because one can conveniently take several cortisol-level readings over a 24-hour period to establish their adrenal hormone rhythms.

Saliva testing has been researched and found to be very accurate for detecting adrenal disorders, in fact it is used to monitor hormone levels in medical research studies, including that done by the World Health Organization. It is also an approved form of testing, by many major health insurance companies, such as Blue Cross/Blue Shield. Many pharmacies carry the type manufactured by "ZRT Labs, Inc.", which is also an approved blood lab, so one can check with their local pharmacy to see if they carry this brand, should they wish to test their adrenal function.

Most adrenal saliva tests are not expensive and can be highly-diagnostic in detecting states of adrenal fatigue in people who are presenting with the symptoms of this common syndrome that is associated with chronic stress and that is more common in people suffering from other chronic illnesses, including thyroid disorders.

3. Adrenal Fatigue by Any Other Name

Some medical sources state that up to 80% of the general population will experience Adrenal Fatigue at some point during their lives. Understanding this stress-related syndrome, is key to recovery.

Adrenal fatigue is a condition in which a person's stress hormones become imbalanced, with the main problem being a diminished level of cortisol reserves.

"ADRENAL FATIGUE" MEANS LOW CORTISOL HORMONE RESERVES

Cortisol is referred to by medical sources, as "the stress hormone". When a person has experienced a traumatic event, such as a catastrophic accident, the sudden loss of a loved one or an ongoing chronic stressor, such as a highly-stressful job or the onset of a life-changing illness, their adrenal hormones can become exhausted. Once this occurs, they can no longer tolerate stress, even at normal, everyday levels. At this point, they will begin to experience bodily symptoms of low cortisol levels, sometimes also referred to as "hypoadrenia" and "hypercortisolemia".

The Symptoms of Adrenal Fatigue May include:

- feeling stressed-out

- insomnia at nighttime

- daytime sleepiness

- general feeling of illness

- body aches

- depressed mood

- low immune function (easily contracting viruses and allergens)

- chronic fatigue

Many doctors will pronounce a patient "normal" when they pass the typical tests that are usually considered to be the only ones needed to diagnose low adrenal function. These will usually consist of either an "ACTH Stimulation Test" and/or a snapshot blood cortisol reading (one blood draw). The problem is that "Adrenal Fatigue" is a disruption of "cortisol rhythm" (the hormone that helps the body to cope-with and recover from stress) and is not necessarily a problem with cortisol being low all of the time. It also doesn't manifest the same way true, full-blown adrenal insufficiency does, so it is not a problem with the adrenals not being capable of stimulation (most people with Adrenal Fatigue, pass the ACTH 'Stimulation' test).

Subclinical dysfunction of the adrenal glands is not usually found until a multi-reading test is performed to gauge a patient's cortisol rhythm over a 24-hour period (multiple blood or saliva samples, at different points of the day). Even a test that takes two readings, one at morning upon waking when cortisol levels are supposed to be highest and one at midnight when levels are supposed to be lowest, can help give a cortisol average, rather than just a single snapshot level.

LOW CORTISOL ILLNESSESS IN MEDICAL STUDIES

What really convinced me years ago, that mild adrenal dysfunction does exist and that it has been proven in medical research to be a true illness, are the study articles published in regard to syndromes like Chronic Fatigue Syndrome, Fibromyalgia and PTSD (Post Traumatic Stress disorder). These articles clearly state that people with these type syndromes, suffer low cortisol levels and they have also found strong association of these syndromes to chronic stressors, from either prolonged or sudden stressful events.

Here are three medical research article examples:

1. The National Institutes of Health - Centers for Disease Control, conducted a study of Chronic Fatigue Syndrome patients (CFS), some years ago and published a press release on their findings. The study was headed by a "Dr. Straus" and in their conclusions, they state that CFS patients have slightly lower cortisol levels, than do healthy people within the general public. They also stated that even subtle cortisol deficiency causes lethargy and fatigue in affected individuals.

2. In another medical research study, titled "Cortisol and Hypothalamic-Pituitary-Gonadal Axis Hormones", researchers found that the women studied, who were Chronic Fatigue Syndrome patients, had "lower morning cortisol levels", than did the healthy control patients who participated in the study. They also stated that the low cortisol contrasted with elevated cortisol levels, that are typically found in patients with Major Depression.

3. In a study published by The New England Journal of Medicine, titled: "Low Cortisol Levels in Children of Parents with PTSD", it was found that children of Holocaust survivors, seemingly inherited a condition of low cortisol from their parents. The study points out that low cortisol levels are often associated with Post Traumatic Stress Disorder. They found that

these children of people with PTSD, were also experiencing symptoms of the disorder, including mood and anxiety disorders. The low cortisol they found in the study participants, was evident at "several points during a 24-hour period".

While research articles do not use the term "adrenal fatigue", this is exactly what is being described by them. They will instead use terms such as "mild adrenal insufficiency", "Blunted HPA axis", "hypocortisolism" or simply "low cortisol". These type research articles are available out there in significant numbers, so doctors who still do not accept sub-clinical adrenal insufficiency as being a real illness, need to look at a few of these studies.

Adrenal Fatigue by whatever other name they wish to call it, does exist and it is found in a variety of stress-related syndromes.

ADRENAL FATIGUE TREATMENTS

What treatments are available to help patients with Adrenal Fatigue? The more basic treatments are those a person can do with self-effort involving lifestyle changes.

Getting more rest and sleep can be tremendously helpful for fatigued adrenals. Cutting back and even eliminating stimulants from the diet, such as refined sugars, caffeine, alcohol and tobacco, can also help. Reducing stress, through relaxation and pursuit of enjoyable activities that allow for stress-reduction, can help as well. Exercising to your tolerance level, can help build up the adrenals, by strengthening the body in general but exercise must not be overdone but should rather be increased gradually at a safe and helpful pace.

Supplements that can also be very helpful in building up adrenal function, include good multivitamins and other nutrients, including B-12, B6, B5, vitamin C, magnesium and zinc. People with fatigued adrenals can also take short-term over-the-counter hormone-supplements to add to their vitamin regimen, such as DHEA, which is an adrenal hormone, that converts into other needed hormones including the sex ones, if these are also low in the body. Adrenal glandular, which is animal based adrenal extract, containing adrenal gland tissue and that usually also contains licorice root extract, can help the body produce higher levels of cortical (cortisol) -- the major "stress hormone".

I usually strongly caution people however, to take these types of supplements as recommended by the manufacturers of them (found on their product labels), following all their warnings and directions. Also let your doctor know what supplements you decide to take, to make sure he/she doesn't feel they will interact adversely with any treatments you are already taking (contraindications).

MY PERSONAL EXPERIENCE WITH ADRENAL FATIGUE

I the author, have experienced Adrenal Fatigue, that became severe at one point after I experienced the onset of autoimmune thyroid disease (Hashimoto's), which caused me hypothyroidism. My Adrenal Fatigue over time, together with the thyroid disease, caused me to also experience the development of Chronic Fatigue Syndrome (MD diagnosed). Even with thyroid hormone replacement treatments, I must continue working on my adrenal function, to prevent phases of severe adrenal exhaustion from recurring.

Repeated tests I had ordered in the past, by my treating doctors, to check my adrenal hormone levels, revealed very low cortical levels for over a year period of time (also called "cortical"), in fact some of these readings were clinically low -- sometimes coming very close to meeting the definition for "Adrenal Insufficiency". I did, however, pass an "ACTH Stimulation test", ruling out true "Addison's disease" (irreversible adrenal gland damage). Even Medical Doctors looking at these test results, admitted that my cortical was very low but some of them told me that there was no treatment available for hypocortisolemia (another term for the condition), unless Addison's disease was definitively diagnosed.

I began using the treatments I have listed above, and I began to see significant improvement, which I maintain to this day. I now only take a good multi-vitamin, having weaned off the other adrenal supplements, plus I do continue to take medication for hypothyroidism -- "Armour Thyroid", natural hormone replacement medication (MD prescribed). I continue to take caution because overwork, too much stress and inadequate rest/sleep, can result in adrenal setbacks for me. However, I seldom experience setbacks as severely or as often as I did before I could understand the cause and implementing treatments.

SEE YOUR DOCTOR

If you feel you may be suffering from Adrenal Fatigue, talk to your Doctor about it. You might even consider seeing a Holistic MD or an Osteopath Doctor, because these types of physicians often recognize this stress-related syndrome, more often than do other types of medical doctors.

4. Adrenal Fatigue can Hinder Hypothyroid Treatment

For many thyroid patients on hormone replacement treatment for their hypothyroidism, the results can be less than satisfactory and for others, it can be downright disappointing however, for a percentage of treated patients, results can be very successful. With this said, I will now discuss a seldom-recognized problem of "worsening adrenal fatigue", in hypothyroid patients who have the condition and see it increase in severity, when they receive thyroid hormones into their systems.

There are many factors that can hinder the effectiveness of thyroid hormone replacement treatment but in this chapter, we will look at one of the more common problems that is experienced by patients -- called "adrenal fatigue". It is always my intention when addressing such a subject, to avoid any negative references to medical professionals, out of concern that such discussion will appear to be directed at all who are in these areas of medical fields, so let me say emphatically, that this is not my intention in this article either! There are many excellent medical professionals out there but there are also those who for some reason are not as well-informed as others or who are not as updated on advancements in treatments as other doctors are.

One common problem that hypothyroid patients experience, is co-existing "adrenal fatigue" (sub-clinical adrenal insufficiency), which can result in a negative affect for a period, from the introduction of thyroid hormone replacement medication into their systems. The main hormone adrenal fatigue patients are low on, is "cortisol", the stress hormone that helps the body to cope with stressors both physical and mental (hypocortisolemia). Cortisol is also essential in its role in giving our bodies the ability to metabolize thyroid hormone and in dealing with the added stress to the body from increased levels of thyroid hormone being introduced into it, via hormone replacement medication.

The manufacturers of thyroid medications themselves, acknowledge in their "contraindications" notices, that patients with "untreated adrenal cortical insufficiency", can experience a worsening of their low-adrenal state, if they implement thyroid hormone replacement medication without correcting any existing adrenal insufficiency. This in my opinion is the very reason many thyroid patients experience a worsening of symptoms, for a period, when they begin thyroid hormone medication treatment. They may also at times experience a re-surge of their symptoms, if adrenal fatigue (mild adrenal insufficiency) tends to return from time to time.

These patients have a sub-clinical form of adrenal insufficiency, due to slow developing hypothyroidism or long-standing hypothyroidism and the introduction of thyroid hormone into their systems, causes an immediate worsening of their adrenal fatigue (Note: This does not occur in all hypothyroid patients.). Certain symptoms will worsen, just as stated by the pharmaceutical companies who make thyroid hormone medications. They further state that if the adrenal insufficiency is full-blown (much rarer), the patient can experience an "adrenal crises ", which is a medical emergency that can result in coma or death. This more-severe response does not happen to patients who have the more common adrenal fatigue and not full-blown adrenal insufficiency, but their symptoms can still be concerning and significant.

The problem with this scenario, is that many doctors do not recognize sub-clinical forms of adrenal insufficiency (adrenal fatigue) and therefore, a patient who experiences a worsening of symptoms when starting thyroid medication, are either told it is in their head (imagined) or not thyroid related but from another cause. An increase in joint pain they may be told, is co-existing arthritis. The increase in fatigue and emotional symptoms, they may be told is an emotional issue needing an antidepressant. The possibilities could very well happen apart from any adrenal fatigue. However, the fact that these symptoms increase after starting thyroid medication, is in my opinion, a reaction that merits further investigation by the patient's doctor, not to exclude tests to see if their adrenal hormones might be the culprit.

It is my understanding that physician references, used by Doctors, recommend testing patients for possible low-adrenal function, before starting them on thyroid hormone medication however, this is seldom done. My belief is that this is true, that full-blown adrenal insufficiency is quite rare. The problem is however, that those who have a sub-clinical form that still causes a negative reaction from implementing thyroid medication, are left to suffer until their own adrenals slowly recover on their own, or until they add some adrenal support to their regimen, to help them recover.

The two questions I would pose to anyone in the medical field who believe adrenal fatigue is not a real condition would be these:

1. If hypothyroidism causes a slowing down of all bodily functions and organs, how could it not be possible that the adrenals would also be greatly affected in some patients?

2. Why, if sub-clinical hypothyroidism is recognized and pre-diabetes (insulin resistance) and other sub-clinical organ dysfunctions are recognized, that this is not also the case with low adrenal function?

By simply getting adrenal hormone levels tested, adrenal fatigue can be seen plainly in black and white on lab results. The problem is, these patients with low adrenal hormone levels, such as cortical/cortisol, will usually pass a test that is recognized by many doctors, as the only true test of adrenal function, called the "ACTH Stimulation Test". If a patient has a negative (good) result from this test, which certainly is diagnostic of full-blown adrenal dysfunction, many doctors will look no further. This leaves the patient with sub-clinical adrenal hypofunction, with no further options for resolving their problem.

It is my opinion that even when a patient passes an ACTH Stimulation test but their actual adrenal hormones are still revealed to be low on lab results, how could it possibly hurt to treat this condition with some of the non-steroidal treatments that are available (most being as safe as a daily multivitamin)? The only treatment for true, full-blown adrenal insufficiency, is lifelong corticosteroid steroids (e.g. Prednisone and Cortef) and there are actually some doctors who will use these steroids to treat severe adrenal fatigue, under strict control and for short-term until the patient's adrenal function is restored to normal (afterward they will take non-prescription adrenal supplements). There are, however, non-steroid treatments that are safer and have proven to be very effective in helping restore adrenal function, in patients with adrenal fatigue. Once this is accomplished, these patients have much better improvement from their thyroid hormone replacement treatment! If the thyroid hormone medication manufacturers recognize this problem as being a real possibility, it should always be a consideration, when a thyroid patient has a negative reaction to thyroid hormone replacement therapy.

5. Adrenal Fatigue Gaining Recognition

For many years, the syndrome of "Adrenal Fatigue" has been largely unrecognized. In the past, doctors typically only recognized the more serious adrenal conditions -- the ones classified as diseases, rather than syndromes. They are understandably more concerned about conditions that cause full-blown "adrenal insufficiency". The main disease that is in this category, is called "Addison's Disease", which can be very severe and even life-threatening if treatment is not administered to control it. These forms of full-blown adrenal insufficiency are not "stress-caused" syndromes, as Adrenal Fatigue is, but they are caused by diseased organs (damaged adrenal glands that are failing). They are often irreversible, unlike a "fatigued adrenal state" which is most-often reversible with proper treatment and ongoing care.

Conditions that can negatively influence or contribute to Adrenal Fatigue, causing it to worsen or to occur more frequently, include Thyroid Diseases, Anxiety Disorders (PTSD is a major one) and other diseases that either seriously affect the body or cause a great deal of mental and emotional stress. It is also my opinion, coming from a great deal of search/research on the subject, that both CFS (Chronic Fatigue Syndrome) and FMS (Fibromyalgia Syndrome), are conditions that are strongly related to Adrenal Fatigue. This has also been concluded by medical research studies, including those that have been undertaken by the U.S. National Institutes of Health (abstracts of these studies can be found on the "PubMed" website).

My question to those who still do not recognize the reality of Adrenal Fatigue, would be this; "If other organs of the body become fatigued, from relentless overuse of them, how could the adrenals escape this same reaction, when bombarded with chronic, prolonged stress?"

People suffering Adrenal Fatigue, are tested many times for levels of cortical/cortisol (the "stress Hormone") and are found to have very low-normal levels and even clinically low levels. They will, however, usually pass the "ACTH Stimulation test" -- the one most often used to detect severe adrenal diseases and one that can rule out true adrenal insufficiency. It is sometimes concluded that patients need no treatment when they do not have full blown adrenal hypofunction (overt hypoadrenia). This, in my opinion is a disservice to patients, who suffer very real symptoms from Adrenal Fatigue syndromes.

6. Adrenal Fatigue is Medically Confirmed

What I endeavor to point out about medical research articles I cite in my own articles on the Adrenal Fatigue subject, is how clearly, they recognize mild types of low adrenal function. One of these articles, found on the PubMed website (National Institutes of Health/National Library of Medicine), is among many that recognize Adrenal Fatigue type syndromes. The title of the article: "Stress-induced hypocortisolemia diagnosed as psychiatric disorders responsive to hydrocortisone replacement."

This online abstract, which can be found by using the title of it in a Google search, states that people can develop states of low adrenal cortisol levels (insufficient levels of the "stress hormone"),in later life, if they experience early life traumatic stress. The article goes on to state that treatment of the condition with hydrocortisone therapy (synthetic cortisol steroid treatments), brought relief of post traumatic emotional and physical symptoms, being experienced by the study participants who had fatigued adrenals.

The article is among many others that conclude that "stress" can be the cause of hypocortisolemia, cortisol being the adrenal hormone that moderates stress in the body but that becomes inadequate with Adrenal Fatigue syndromes. This is why I refer to Adrenal Fatigue as a "stress syndrome". Ongoing stress (chronic) can have the very same effect in taxing the adrenals as do sudden traumatic experiences (Post Traumatic Stress). Despite the obvious, there are still some in the medical community who deny the existence of Adrenal Fatigue conditions. Are they overlooking dozens of medical research conclusions? They are in fact overlooking them.

For many years, medical research sources that address the Adrenal Fatigue subject (though usually referred to by other names), point out that chronic stress first elevates cortisol but prolonged demand for this added cortisol output, eventually exhausts/fatigues the adrenals and cortisol levels begin to deplete. Another interesting PubMed article has also been published, that points out this very fact regarding cortisol first remaining high and eventually falling to suppressed levels. The one I refer to is titled: "Low cortisol production in chronic stress. The connection stress-somatic disease is a challenge for future research".

These articles give a perfect description of what happens with Adrenal Fatigue syndromes and yet some physicians within the medical community seem to be overlooking the obvious. The best thing that we who are patient advocates can do for the time being, is to continue informing the public about Adrenal Fatigue Syndromes, until there is more widespread acknowledgment of this very real illness that can be treated successfully.

7. Adrenal Fatigue Steroid Treatment

People suffering chronic Adrenal Fatigue (frequent or ongoing), will often diligently seek a treatment that will provide them relief for their concerning symptoms. For many, the option of "cortisol replacement therapy" is seriously considered and some patients find physicians willing to give them a trial of the treatment. Glucocorticoids, which are synthetic cortisol replacement drugs, are steroids that require caution when used to treat adrenal disorders or health conditions of any kind. (NOTE: This is not an ant-cortisol article but simply one that advises caution to Adrenal Fatigue patients who are considering implementing a cortisol therapy of any type.)

Steroid cortisol supplementation requires a qualified physician in most cases. While some cases of Adrenal Fatigue have been successfully treated using synthetic cortisol steroids (hydrocortisone), other cases result in further suppression of the adrenal glands by the treatment. In some cases, this may be due to the dose not being monitored closely or not being dosed correctly (incorrect dose amounts). It is of most importance that this type treatment is administered by a qualified medical professional, who is knowledgeable in adrenal hormone replacement therapies. The physician would also need to be skilled in monitoring a patient's hormone levels while they are being treated. A patient considering the treatment should also be thoroughly informed about the possible risks and side effects.

Hydro-cortisone therapy in CFS patients with low cortisol levels yielded some interesting results. In the year 1996, the U.S. National Institutes of Health (NIH) – Centers for Disease Control, conducted studies of Chronic Fatigue Syndrome patients, treating them with doses of hydrocortisone (synthetic cortisol) to replace sub-clinically low cortisol levels. The trial of cortisol replacement therapy followed other studies that found low cortisol levels in CFS patients compared to healthy controls (non-CFS participants). The study was an attempt to see if the cortisol supplementation would relieve CFS symptoms.

Over-replacing cortisol can cause the adrenal glands to shut down. The NIH study of cortisol supplementation in CFS patients concluded that in some of the participants, the drug significantly relieved their symptoms but an adverse effect of "adrenal suppression" (further decrease in adrenal cortical output) was seen in some of them after several weeks on the drug. This resulted in the conclusion that cortisol supplementation was not a safe treatment due to the risk of the treatment causing significant adrenal insufficiency. The outcome of the trial may have been more favorable if lower doses had been administered because CFS patients have mild adrenal insufficiency and do not require full cortisol replacement as do those with full-blown adrenal insufficiency.

This study was revealing and the facts it presents, should be given serious consideration by Adrenal Fatigue patients who are considering cortisol replacement therapy.

8. CFS Fibromyalgia and Low Cortisol

For more than ten years, researchers studying Chronic Fatigue Syndrome (CFS) and Fibromyalgia Syndrome, have conducted studies regarding adrenal function in patients with these syndromes. They have concluded that patients are found to be experiencing "low adrenal function" as one of the features of these syndromes. This co-existing condition is also called "adrenal fatigue", "adrenal exhaustion" and "low adrenal reserve". Reputable medical sources also state that patients with thyroid disease are at more risk than the general population, for also having co-existing CFS and/or Fibromyalgia (FMS).

Through testing of a patient's adrenal hormones, it can be determined if that person has low-functioning adrenals. In addition to blood testing, saliva tests are also accurate for testing the "free levels" of adrenal hormones, the main ones being DHEA and cortisol. A "24-hour urinary cortisol test", can also be done, to test adrenal-cortisol levels.

Another major adrenal function blood test is also available, called the "ACTH Stimulation Test". This one is designed to confirm or rule out true "adrenal insufficiency" (full blown). Most CFS and Fibromyalgia patients do not have true, full blown adrenal insufficiency but a milder form of adrenal fatigue/exhaustion.

Research conclusions by major Medical Research groups, including the NIH, state that low cortical/cortisol levels are found to be a contributing factor in CFS/FMS, due to dysfunction of the HPA Axis (Hypothalamus-Pituitary-Adrenal Axis -- the major endocrine brain glands). It is my opinion because of this, that CFS/FMS has as one of its features, a form of adrenal fatigue, that does not meet the definition for true "adrenal insufficiency" and because of this, it cannot be medically treated the same.

With full blown adrenal insufficiency, low adrenal hormones must be replaced through steroid treatment (cortisone-steroid/hydrocortisone). With lesser forms of low adrenal function, such as adrenal fatigue, steroid treatment can possibly worsen the adrenal problem because it can cause "adrenal suppression". This means a patient may have to take the steroids for the rest of their life because anything less than very short-term use of them, can cause this suppression of the adrenal glands. The point being that only patients with true adrenal insufficiency, should be replaced with long-term and usually lifelong steroid cortisol replacement therapy.

Adrenal fatigue is a milder condition, usually caused by traumatic or chronic stress. This, as opposed to an overtly worsening condition, from diseased or damaged adrenal glands or what is referred to as "Addison's disease" (another name for true, full-blown adrenal insufficiency).

9. Common Adrenal Fatigue Treatments

Adrenal Fatigue is a common complaint in thyroid patients.

Testing cortisol levels is important when adrenal hormone imbalance is suspected because of symptoms like fatigue, cravings for stimulants (e.g. the need for more coffee and refined sugars) and a diminishing tolerance for stress (feeling stressed out). It becomes even more important when a condition like Adrenal Fatigue is being treated because retests (whether by blood or saliva), are the only way to monitor the effectiveness of a self-administered treatment.

When doctors are treating patients for hormonal imbalances, they order retests every few weeks at first, until they see how an established dose of hormone therapy is going in a patient's body. Afterward, they may only have to retest every few months to monitor a treatment. If a patient manifests serious side effects at any point during a treatment, doctors will usually order a retest right away, as a precaution against increasingly serious complications. Patients who self-administer non-prescription hormone replacement or hormone-raising treatments, should take the same precautions and the same type of retesting schedule, if possible.

With the potential risks involved with use of cortisol supplements, also called "cortical" (those containing cortisol hormone), which includes increased risk for hypertension and elevated glucose levels (high blood sugar), Adrenal Fatigue patients should first consider natural methods for increasing cortisol levels safely.

There are several potential causes for sub-clinically low adrenal function, including Chronic Fatigue Syndrome, Fibromyalgia, chronic and inflammatory diseases, traumatic stress and emotional disorders (depressive disorders and Post Traumatic Stress disorder are known to affect cortisol levels). These conditions can however first result in increased cortisol levels before causing a significant drop in them. Some sources that post information on Adrenal Fatigue Syndromes, refer to the period of increased cortisol levels as "the alarm phase" and the following drop in levels once the adrenals become severely fatigued, they refer to as "the exhaustion phase" (a mid-stage in which symptoms are milder, they call the "resistance response phase").

These facts point to the importance in first testing adrenal cortisol, to determine its level before assuming it to be low and in need of being increased. If borderline low or sub-clinically low levels are not found, then boosting cortisol levels might not be needed. However, test results may reveal the need for adrenal support supplements that help raise cortisol in the body. If supplements are taken to improve adrenal function, it is also important to retest adrenal hormone levels at regular intervals to monitor the treatment.

There are natural methods for increasing cortisol levels. Taking safe over-the-counter supplements that help strengthen fatigued adrenal glands is recommended as a first line of treatment, rather than resorting to cortisol steroids that pose potential risks. Supplements that specifically help boost the adrenals in producing more cortisol, would be "glycyrrhizic acid" which is found in licorice root extract products and "adrenal glandular" which is found in products processed from the adrenal glands of animals, which are usually made from bovine source (beef/cow adrenal glands). Most adrenal glandular products are 'hormone free' however one brand available called "Isocort", contains trace amounts of cortisol in the pellets that are processed from the adrenal glands of New Zealand sheep.

According to sources reporting research on vitamins that help to strengthen fatigued adrenals, vitamins C, B5, B6 and B12 all fall within that category. In some cases, vitamins can be purchased containing all of these stress-helping nutrients, in one daily pill. Those labeled "All B With C" for example or those that are marketed for Adrenal Fatigue relief and contain additional ingredients, such as the brand I sometimes take called "Cortico B5 - B6" (made by the Metagenics Company). Sometimes, a patient with fatigued or exhausted adrenals, will simply have to conduct trial dosing periods, to see which supplement(s) works best for them (4 to 6 weeks will usually reveal progress or failure). As with many health conditions, "patient individuality" can also be a factor in zeroing-in on what works best.

It is recommended that any supplement always be taken at the manufacturer's recommended-dose (instruction labels) and that any supplement is approved by a physician who knows a patient's medical background.

10. Fatigued Adrenals During Hypothyroid Treatment

Adrenal Fatigue can become somewhat of a dilemma for thyroid patients. Medical sources including thyroid hormone medication manufacturers warn that "untreated adrenal cortical insufficiency" (low cortisol) can be worsened by treating hypothyroidism with hormone replacement therapy, without first correcting it or by treating them both simultaneously. What then becomes a question is: "How bad does the low cortisol have to be, to present a real problem?"

Certainly full blown adrenal insufficiency can present with this problem that is warned about but it only takes common sense to realize that adrenal fatigue (subclinical adrenal insufficiency) or adrenal exhaustion (adrenal fatigue that borders on overt adrenal failure) can be negatively-affected by thyroid hormone replacement as well. These are conditions of low cortisol, that are less severe than true adrenal disease (Addison's disease) but that should be considered as potential "opposing factors" in hypothyroid therapies.

Less severe adrenal fatigue, will many times resolve spontaneously when hypothyroidism is corrected because a low functioning thyroid gland causes everything else in the body, including the adrenals, to operate low (the slowed metabolism is systemic - body wide). When adrenal fatigue in hypothyroid patients isn't severe, it usually corrects on its own when hypothyroidism is corrected, and bodily metabolism is restored.

Other patients aren't so fortunate, and you can find their testimonials online, via their blogs and forum posts. They report having struggled with their adrenal fatigue worsening, when they started thyroid hormone medication and that continues to present them with a struggle, as their hypothyroidism is treated as an ongoing therapy. Some of these patients report having intermittent flares of adrenal fatigue, while others report theirs to be chronic and ongoing, with worsening flares occurring easily with stress or with physical exertion. They report that this will be the case with them, even while they are on optimal thyroid hormone therapy.

I personally fit into the category of experiencing intermittent flares of adrenal fatigue. I also experienced a variety of low adrenal symptoms, that worsened with the start of thyroid hormone medication. I feel it's possible that many of the patients, who report worsening symptoms for a while after starting thyroid hormone replacement therapy, may very well be experiencing "adjustment symptoms" as both their thyroid and adrenal hormones are trying to correct to normal levels.

Those patients who seem to never reach a well-adjusted state on thyroid hormone replacement, should have their adrenal hormones blood tested, to see if they have a significant low adrenal hormone problem (insufficient cortisol levels). If this does prove to be the case, their doctors could then adjust their hormone therapy, to include supporting the adrenal glands or they could refer patients to endocrinologists, who specialize in the simultaneous treatment of combined thyroid-adrenal hormone deficiencies.

11. Low Adrenal Function in CFS and FMS

Adrenal Fatigue is a sub-clinical form of adrenal insufficiency, but it is still not recognized widely by the medical community. Certain types of doctors recognize the disorder more than others, including MDs who practice holistic treatments, Naturopaths and Osteopathic Physicians. This condition is also referred to as one of "low adrenal reserves" and "adrenal exhaustion". The condition causes mild to moderate chronic fatigue and reduced stress tolerance (ongoing fatigue and constantly feeling stressed out). Some medical sources are stating that when the condition is prolonged and not treated, through proper rest, improved diet, adrenal-boosting natural supplements and reducing contributing stressors, it may result in the condition becoming a precursor (a pre-condition) to CFS and FMS. I will address these two syndromes that often accompany fatigued adrenals, following below.

Chronic Fatigue Syndrome (CFS):

This condition has also been found to cause a low level of the stress hormone cortisol, evidenced by analyzing the blood and urine cortisol levels in people who experience the illness. Research studies on CFS have repeatedly confirmed this fact and have also found that many patients report that they were experiencing chronic or sudden severe stress just before the onset of the illness. This would mean that CFS is very-possibly also a stress-related condition that causes the adrenal hormone regulating glands in the body to become blunted. The U.S. National Institutes of Health released a report in October of 1996, in which they found through a controlled study, that cortisol supplementation/replacement in patients with CFS had a benefit but was found to be short-lived. Afterward, some patients began experiencing a more severe form of adrenal suppression, meaning it caused a worsening of their adrenal insufficiency after a few weeks on the cortisol replacement drug.

Fibromyalgia Syndrome (FMS):

Being very similar to CFS, Fibromyalgia also has chronic fatigue as a major symptom. The aspect that sets this illness apart from CFS, is the widespread body pain that is not found to be as prominent in CFS patients. Despite this fact, researchers studying both illnesses have found them to have 75% crossover similarities. This includes the fact that FMS patients often report chronic stress as being a factor in their development of the illness.

Several research studies have also found cortisol levels to be low in FMS patients and controlled trials of cortisol supplementation have been conducted to determine if there would be a benefit for these patients. The findings were like those found when supplementing CFS patients with cortisol hormone replacement. While some patients improved, the long-term risks for using the drug did not merit establishing it as a medically recognized treatment for FMS. While the two conditions listed above are commonly found to cause or be co-morbid to mild adrenal insufficiency, other conditions can also be a cause or contributing factor, including other chronic and inflammatory diseases that contribute to increased stress levels in the body.

See a professional, licensed physician for a complete evaluation if you suspect that you may be suffering from a health condition causing mild adrenal insufficiency (Adrenal Fatigue).

12. Prescribed and Natural Adrenal Fatigue Treatment

Over the past few years, I've corresponded with thyroid patients who also suffer severe co-occurring "Adrenal Fatigue". They report that some of their doctors have placed them on a corticosteroid. This is a steroid form of cortisol, to help increase their own levels of this adrenal hormone that becomes low with Adrenal Fatigue. Cortisol is the "stress hormone" that is essential to our bodies for everyday functioning and in coping with everyday stressors. In Adrenal Fatigue patients, the trick in using safe non-steroid supplements, is to strengthen one's own adrenal glands, so that they function better in producing cortisol and other important adrenal hormones. With the more severe "Adrenal Insufficiency" (full blown), patients must be treated with a corticosteroid steroid, to replace the low cortisol.

Some patient's cases are more complicated because some develop Cushing's' Disease from the prolonged use of the adrenal steroids (symptoms of overactive adrenal glands) or they are on the verge of developing it. In cases like these, they have to be tapered off of their corticosteroid drug (e.g. the most common brands being Cortef or Prednisone), very slowly and if while doing so, their cortisol drops down to adrenal insufficiency level, they have to be bumped back up on their dose again and they will possibly have to take the cortisol steroid for the rest of their lives. If at any point a patient develops symptoms of swelling (edema), increased appetite and weight gain, these can be symptoms of having abnormally high cortisol levels, which can cause cushingoid symptoms.

When patients are placed on corticosteroids, they need follow-up blood testing and/or urine testing of their cortisol levels, at regular intervals, like how thyroid hormone therapy is monitored, every two to three months with blood retests. If this isn't done, they can potentially develop symptoms of Cushing's' Disease. I do have other articles online regarding treating Adrenal Fatigue and I don't recommend treating it with corticosteroids (cortisol steroids), whether it's the synthetic type like Prednisone or the more natural Cortef brand. The reason I don't recommend it, is for the very reasons I have stated.

Another reason steroid treatment for Adrenal Fatigue, is not recommended, is due to the possibility of it progressing to full blown Adrenal Insufficiency. Studies by the National Institutes of Health found that treating sub-clinical adrenal insufficiency syndromes, such as Chronic Fatigue Syndrome and Post Traumatic Stress Disorder, can result in further adrenal suppression. Dr. Stephen E. Straus, M.D, who is quoted in a PubMed article states: "Any time long-term steroid therapy is considered, even a low dose, one needs to be concerned that the treatment itself may suppress the adrenal gland's normal production of steroids, which can lead to serious complications." (Quotes from PubMed/NIH, are allowed for public information.)

Some doctors who do treat Adrenal Fatigue with Cortef or Prednisone, will administer it in very small physiological doses and in so doing, can usually avoid complications, with also closely monitoring the patient's cortisol levels via repeat blood testing and by only treating them short-term until their own adrenal glands have improved. Even with this however, it carries a risk and a patient would want to be very confident in their treating Doctor. One cannot suddenly switch from a corticosteroid also called "glucocorticoids", to a simple adrenal support regimen because Adrenal Fatigue support supplements are designed to strengthen a person's own adrenal glands, to begin producing their own adequate amounts of cortisol and most adrenal support, is very safe and can be taken lifelong, like most vitamins and minerals can.

If you are placed on a corticosteroid for Adrenal Fatigue, you'll need close supervision by your Doctor in getting better adjusted on dose or weaned off the medication. It is extremely important that you not try weaning off the medication yourself because this can potentially cause an "adrenal crisis" -- an emergency medical condition that can cause coma or death, if not treated in time.

It wasn't my intention to scare or overly-concern anyone reading this article but rather to point out that corticosteroid treatment is something that takes extreme caution and supervision by a Doctor. You cannot switch from a corticosteroid treatment, to a different type, on your own but you must have a medical professional to help. If you are not confident in your current doctor in supervising your current treatment or in helping you to taper off in discontinuing it, I would certainly recommend seeking the help of another doctor, such as an endocrinologist for a second opinion because steroid treatments of any kind are very serious and you cannot take chances with your health.

13. PTSD Adrenal Insufficiency in Thyroid Patients

Some statistics state that about 10% of people with thyroid disease experience a degree of mild adrenal insufficiency. Mildly insufficient functioning of the adrenals is a condition in which the glands do not produce enough hormones to aid in regulating the body's metabolism, stress coping, inflammation control and sexual functioning. People with sub-normal cortisol levels (the stress-regulating hormone), will often report that they have an ongoing experience with feeling "stressed out". When low levels of cortisol (also called "cortical") are detected in a person, it is sometimes referred to as "hypocortisolemia". Full blown adrenal insufficiency is usually referred to as "Addison's Disease."

There are milder forms of adrenal dysfunction syndromes, which includes "Post Traumatic Stress Disorder" (PTSD), as addressed below:

This condition, abbreviated PTSD, is a traumatic stress-caused condition that is also considered to be an anxiety disorder. People experience the onset of this disorder as a result of severe traumatizing experiences, such as car accidents, acts of violence that are perpetrated upon them, the sudden loss of a loved one or having been in active combat during wartime. The severe shock caused to the body from such incidents, can cause the glands regulating adrenal hormone output to become "blunted", meaning they begin to function at a sub-normal level.

While the adrenal hormones of PTSD sufferers may remain within normal limits, they will be at low or lowest normal (borderline low), which causes them to have a diminished ability to cope with stressors. Research studies on PTSD that are published by reputable medical groups (including the U.S. National Institutes of Health) state that low cortisol levels found in patients with this disorder contributes to their symptoms of anxiety, insomnia and flashbacks, meaning they may mentally relive their traumatic experiences repeatedly.

In controlled test studies, using cortisol supplementation to treat PTSD patients, results showed that symptoms were reduced significantly by carefully monitored physiological dosing to increase their level of the low stress hormone. In other words, the cortical-steroid treatments were administered by medical professionals, with careful monitoring of the participating patient's blood hormone levels. Certainly, a significant percent of thyroid patients, are suffering from this co-morbid condition, many of them being veteran soldiers of foreign wars.

14. Taking Precautions with Adrenal Supplements

Adrenal support, over-the-counter supplements, like adrenal cortex glandular, DHEA and licorice root extract, are not steroids but they have the same end-result of causing fatigued adrenals, to produce their own needed cortisol (what hydrocortisone steroids replace automatically). Patients do need to research adrenal supplements and study the manufacturer's recommendations before using them. It's even better if your doctor is behind you in taking them and monitoring your progress and for observing possible, unwanted side effects.

Much of the medical community, for reasons I cannot understand are reluctant to recognize adrenal support as treatment for adrenal fatigue, possibly because it is not a prescribed treatment or because it is not lab-developed or synthetic but instead, a natural treatment. Who knows for sure why some of them don't pay attention to studies stating the existence of sub-clinical hypoadrenalism, by very reputable groups, including the U.S.-NIH, which found low cortical levels in syndromes like CFS, Fibromyalgia and PTSD? Although these studies go back many years, confirming the existence of subclinical adrenal insufficiency, many still do not recognize it as a real illness.

Since there are other hormone imbalances and conditions that have similar symptoms as "Adrenal Fatigue", in my opinion, a person who suspects they may have a type of the syndrome, should be tested to see where their adrenal hormone levels are (mainly the daytime cortisol rhythm).

Keep in mind as stated above, that many doctors do not recognize adrenal fatigue but only the more severe types of adrenal hypofunction, usually classified as "Addison's Disease". Because of this, they will believe that a patient who passes a test called the "ACTH Stimulation Test", which is designed to detect full blown adrenal insufficiency, needs no further investigation. However, adrenal fatigue is sub-clinical (milder) condition and yet can still cause significant symptoms. A patient with adrenal fatigue will usually pass this test. What they need tested however, are the "free levels" of major adrenal hormones, namely "DHEA & Cortisol", at several points during a 24-hour period.

The ACTH Stimulation Test gauges the adrenals reaction to being stimulated by the pituitary hormone ACTH. The problem is, however, that with Adrenal Fatigue, the adrenals can be stimulated and react, but they still produce low levels of adrenal hormones consistently throughout the day and they usually crash afterward from extra stimulation because adrenal reserves are low. Being stimulated chemically from the outside as opposed having ongoing reserves throughout daytime hours (during main activities), are not the same thing.

Adrenal fatigue and the other syndromes that have adrenal fatigue as a feature of them, have as one proposed cause, a blunted HPA Axis. This is referring to the group of endocrine glands that supply our bodies with needed hormones, as they work in a loop. These glands are the Hypothalamus, Pituitary and Adrenals --- working in sync (axis) with each other. In these adrenal fatigue type disorders, response by these glands becomes "blunted" (slowed down), according to medical research that has been conducted. This is found commonly in conditions like CFS and Fibromyalgia. While some within the medical community believe this to be a bogus idea, there are U.S. Gov/NIH medical studies to back it the existence of subclinical hypoadrenia (published on their "PubMed" website). Because of this fact, adrenal fatigue syndromes should be looked at as real illnesses, with reputable medical research behind the existence of them!

Many medical Doctors do not seem to be aware of these findings as mentioned above but it is referred to by several departments of the National Institutes of Health, including the CDC, NIAMS and The American Journal of Psychiatry. People who suspect that they have sub-clinically low adrenal function, can obtain saliva home test kits, inexpensively, that test the major adrenal hormones (cortisol and DHEA). One can Check with their local Pharmacy and if the test kits aren't carried by them, the tests can be ordered online.

If you test your adrenal hormones and see that they are consistently low-normal, near borderline or even clinically low, it would be time to check into adrenal support. You could first see if you can obtain supplements through your doctor, who will most likely want to first order tests to make sure you don't have full-blown adrenal insufficiency. If it is found that you are only suffering from a milder case of Adrenal Fatigue and not from actual adrenal disease causing you to develop full-blown adrenal insufficiency, your treatment option becomes clear. If your doctor doesn't believe in treating lesser forms of low-adrenal function, you might try finding an osteopath or naturopath physician, who does recognize adrenal fatigue and the available treatments for it.

If these avenues are not available, you may want to purchase over-the-counter adrenal support supplements and to treat yourself. Should you do this, I would of course recommend taking only the manufacturer's recommended doses and that you do research on the support supplements you may choose to take. This is to make sure they are safe for you and that there are no contraindications that might affect you -- meaning they will not interact negatively with any other treatments you may already be taking for other health issues.

Adrenal support at manufacturer's recommended doses, are usually as safe as daily vitamins but taking added precautions is always the wise thing to do, to protect yourself from even the smallest possibility of adverse or allergic reactions to adrenal boosting supplements.

15. Treatable Fatigued Adrenals in Chronic Illnesses

Some sources reporting on syndromes of sub clinically low adrenal function, are reporting that at least 10% of thyroid patients will develop cases of "Adrenal Fatigue". There are other illnesses and syndromes that are associated with mild adrenal dysfunction as well, including Chronic Fatigue Syndrome (CFS), Fibromyalgia and Post Traumatic Stress Disorder. Medical research studies have also shown that patients with diseases such as Rheumatoid Arthritis and Chronic Inflammatory Bowel Disease, have also been found to have a significant lowering of adrenal hormones.

The milder form of low adrenal function is treated many times with supplements such as DHEA, Adrenal Glandular and multi-vitamins that contain those that help boost adrenal function (vitamins C, B5 and B6), as well as B-12 shots. These are all over-the-counter supplements, except for B-12 shots but you can also purchase B-12 in oral, over-the-counter form. All these supplements have been found to be helpful in resolving Adrenal Fatigue conditions that make sufferers feel fatigued and stressed out.

Things medical researchers have studied in regard to CFS and Fibromyalgia for example, are the facts that these syndromes can have different triggers for different patients but for many, it is an underlying viral, autoimmune or bacterial type infection in the body, that causes chronic activation of the immune system. Over time, this uses-up some of the stress hormone reserves because the adrenal glands have a major role in releasing cortisol, the body's natural anti-inflammatory, to help moderate and to ward off inflammation.

Cortisol (also called "cortical"), is the main "stress hormone", that helps the body to deal with stressors of all kinds. Without it, even the smallest stressor would cause shock and death (an adrenal crises). It, along with adrenaline, are classified as "fight or flight" hormones that help protect the body from the effects of anything including minor emotional stress-events, to major traumatic occurrences such as a car accident or a serious, life-threatening disease.

This in my opinion is why persons with CFS/FMS have such low tolerance for stressors both emotional and physical. With low adrenal function, even mild emotional and physical stressors can result in major fatigue and a feeling of being "stressed out". This coupled with the immune system dysfunction that CFS/FMS patients are also reported to have, and you have syndromes that manifest with seriously significant symptoms. It may be that the immune deficiency found in both CFS and Fibromyalgia is also a type of burn-out involving the adrenal system, due to constant, ongoing activation of it, that the body eventually loses the ability to continue.

As with all other opinions about CFS and Fibromyalgia, we have to consider all of the above, as some of the many theories and facts that are out there, however, I feel that the evidence for low adrenal function in CFS and Fibromyalgia, is overwhelming. What I have described, is what I feel connects these syndromes to a form of adrenal fatigue, which continues to be a controversial illness that many MDs refuse to acknowledge. Over time however, I believe adrenal syndromes will gain wider recognition. In the meantime, we who work at being "patient advocates" on behalf of adrenal syndrome sufferers, will continue to help inform the public about these illnesses, to the best of our abilities.

16. Treating Adrenal Fatigue

What treatments are available to help patients with Adrenal Fatigue? The more basic treatments are those a person can do with self-effort involving lifestyle changes. Getting more rest and sleep can be tremendously helpful for fatigued adrenals. Cutting back and even eliminating stimulants from the diet, such as refined sugars, caffeine, alcohol and tobacco, can also help. Reducing stress, through relaxation and pursuit of enjoyable activities that allow for stress-reduction, can help as well. Exercising to your tolerance level, can help build up the adrenals, by strengthening the body in general but exercise must not be overdone but should rather be increased gradually at a safe and helpful pace.

Supplements that can also be very helpful in building up adrenal function, include good multivitamins, the "B" vitamins (especially B-12, B6 and B5), vitamin C, magnesium and zinc. People with fatigued adrenals can also take short-term over-the-counter supplements to add to their vitamin regimen, such as DHEA, which is an adrenal hormone, that will convert into other needed hormones including the sex ones, if these are low in the body. Adrenal glandular, which is animal based adrenal extract, containing adrenal gland tissue and licorice root extract, can help the body produce higher levels of cortical (cortisol) -- the major "stress hormone". I usually strongly caution people however, to take these types of supplements as recommended by the manufacturers of them (found on their product labels), following all of their warnings and directions. Also let your doctor know what supplements you decide to take, to make sure she doesn't feel they will interact adversely with any treatments you are already taking (contraindications).

I the author, have experienced Adrenal Fatigue, that became severe at one point after I experienced the onset of autoimmune thyroid disease (Hashimoto's), which caused me hypothyroidism. My Adrenal Fatigue over time, together with the thyroid disease, caused me to also experience the development of Chronic Fatigue Syndrome (MD diagnosed). Even with thyroid hormone replacement treatments, I have had to continue working on my adrenal function, to prevent phases of severe adrenal exhaustion from occurring. Repeated tests I had ordered by my treating doctors, to check my adrenal hormone levels, revealed very low cortical levels for over a year period of time, in fact some of these readings were clinically low (sometimes meeting the definition for "Adrenal Insufficiency". I did however, pass an ACTH Stimulation test, ruling out true "Addison's disease" (irreversible adrenal gland damage) . Even Medical Doctors looking at these test results, admitted that my cortical was very low but some of them told me that there was no treatment available for it, unless Addison's disease was diagnosed.

I began using the treatments I have listed above and began to see significant improvement, which I maintain to this day. I now only take a good multivitamin, having weaned off the other adrenal supplements, plus I do continue to take medication for hypothyroidism -- "Armour Thyroid", natural hormone replacement medication (MD prescribed). I continue to take caution because overwork, too much stress and inadequate rest/sleep, can result in setbacks for me. However, I seldom experience setbacks as severely or as often as I did before I could understand the cause and implementing treatments. If you feel you may be suffering from Adrenal Fatigue, talk to your Doctor about it. You might even consider seeing a Holistic MD or an Osteopath Doctor, because these types of physicians often recognize this stress-related syndrome.

17. Treating Adrenal Fatigue Naturally or Medically

Hydrocortisone steroids (corticosteroids) can replace low cortisol in people with various types of "adrenal insufficiency" (full blown adrenal failure). Prescribed drugs available for this, include the brand names "Prednisone" and "Cortef" but medical sources warn of the fact that if a doctor is not highly-skilled in administering these drugs for "adrenal fatigue" (subclinical adrenal failure), they can actually worsen it, by causing further adrenal suppression.

True adrenal insufficiency is easier to treat in one sense because patients need full cortisol replacement therapy, as a lifelong treatment, while adrenal fatigue sufferers need "less than full replacement" and only administered for short term. It's possible there is a dose of corticosteroid/cortical/cortisol, that is safe for treating adrenal fatigue with but medical research has yet to find the specific treatment, that will work for a large cross-section of people, safely and with no seriously adverse effects or risks.

If safe over-the-counter supplements can be tried first for mildly low cortisol states, this is a better way to treat adrenal fatigue type conditions. A doctor is needed for corticosteroid treatment, if there is a need for it to be administered as well at some point, for stubborn cases of adrenal fatigue. However, there are helpful over-the-counter supplements for adrenal fatigue including the "B" vitamins, especially B-5, B-6 and B-12, vitamin C, licorice root extract (only as label-recommended and for short term therapy) and processed adrenal glandular supplements (usually beef/bovine source), using the same precautions as with licorice root.

A low maintenance dose of licorice root (an herbal known to help the adrenals manufacture more cortisol) may be stated as being safe on a manufacturer's label and if so, this is likely an accurate statement, at the dose they cite in their directions. People taking the supplement, however, do need to monitor for any hypertensive effects and for tachycardia (rapid resting heart rate) or other possible heart arrhythmia symptoms. As with any natural supplements, one should inform their doctor about taking any of them, as a precaution against them contraindicating their use with other treatments one has already been prescribed (advising against combining them).

Some people report significant improvement while on specially formulated, herbal adrenal support supplements as well, including use of a supplement called "Adreset", made by the Metagenics Company (approximately as safe as a daily vitamin). This company also makes a vitamin supplement for adrenal support called "Cortico B5-B6", containing magnesium and vitamin C in it as well. My own pharmacist recommended these supplements to me because they are pharmaceutical grade and they have helped with my adrenal fatigue flares a great deal.

A company that makes a non-hormone adrenal glandular is "Vitamin Research Product Company" (VRP, Inc.) who offers their product over the counter, called "CortiTrophin". Their company has Pharmacists and MDs behind research and development of their supplements, and therefore I believe they are more reputable than some of the other adrenal supplement manufacturers that are out there. All these natural remedies I have listed, are the self-treatment options we have, if we suffer adrenal fatigue. Much of the medical community has this condition on a back shelf, until it becomes more widely accepted/recognized as a real illness.

Following is a short quote from a PubMed published article (from The U.S.-NIH website), titled: "STRESS-INDUCED HYPO-CORTISOLEMIA DIAGNOSED AS PSYCHIATRIC DISORDERS RESPONSIVE TO HYDROCORTISONE REPLACEMENT" (reprints allowed for public education)

Here is that quote:

"...cortisol deficiency is rarely considered in a medical or psychiatric work-up, so persons with mild to moderate cortisol insufficiency are for the most part relegated to receiving a psychiatric diagnosis when, in fact, the same disorder is represented.

18. Review for Adrenal Fatigue The 21st Century Stress Syndrome

This is my review of Dr. James Wilson's sensational book, covering the common, yet often unrecognized illness called "Adrenal Fatigue". This stress syndrome affects a majority people at some point.

I bought this wonderful book about adrenal fatigue titled "Adrenal Fatigue The 21st Century Stress Syndrome", about two years ago, at a Hastings bookstore. It was very interesting and hard to put down, so I finished it within a couple of days even though it contains over 300 pages of reading. This book is authored by Dr. James L. Wilson, who has a PhD in Human Nutrition, having also completed studies in immunology, microbiology, pharmacology and toxicology. He also has master's degrees in bio-nutrition and psychology and is a Doctor of Chiropractic and Naturopathic Medicine. I was drawn to this book, due to my own experience with adrenal fatigue, which presented with the typical symptoms, that are reported as being experienced by many other adrenal fatigue sufferers, worldwide.

These symptoms include the following:

- fatigue and malaise following even mild physical activity
- body aches and muscle weakness
- a change in sleep patterns (including insomnia)
- dizziness when first standing up
- difficulty concentrating
- increased frequency of headaches
- cravings for salt, sugar and caffeine

- feeling continually "stressed out"

- low immune function (increased viral infections and allergies)

I have dealt with both hypothyroid symptoms and those of adrenal fatigue, for many years and I have learned to tell the differences between them. According to another well-known adrenal fatigue medical researcher - Michael Lam, MD, in his article titled "Adrenal Fatigue versus Hypothyroidism", low thyroid function can develop from longstanding, untreated adrenal fatigue. I know by my own personal experience, that when my hypothyroidism is well-treated, as evident by my blood tests of thyroid hormone levels, any ongoing symptoms I continue to experience are very likely caused by adrenal fatigue. This will require separate treatment and I have seen great results by implementing the treatments recommended in Dr. Wilson's book. The endocrine systems of the body work together (e.g. thyroid, adrenals and pancreas) and when one of these systems is not operating correctly, it can also negatively affect the others. Therefore, I believe Dr. Wilson's book to be an invaluable resource for thyroid patients, as well as for those experiencing adrenal-only problems.

More Medical Doctors are Recognizing Adrenal Fatigue

The Forward for the book was written by Dr. Jonathan V. Wright MD, who cites the fact that there are other MDs who have dedicated time to medical research and helping to inform the medical community about this very real medical condition, including John Tintera MD and William Jeffries MD. These facts are contrasted by the mentions by Dr. Wilson, in which he points out the fact in this book, that many doctors still do not recognize adrenal fatigue and therefore will not test patients for it or recommend treatments. This is changing slowly however, with more doctors beginning to recognize this syndrome as a true illness that can seriously affect the quality-of-life of those who experience it. My own doctor for example, who is a Board-Certified Family Practitioner, fully recognizes this stress syndrome and provides her patients who suffer adrenal fatigue, with sheets that outline some of the treatments recommended by Dr. Wilson in this book.

Stressors are the Major Cause of Adrenal Fatigue

The book helps the reader to understand the importance of normal adrenal function in our everyday lives and then addresses the stressors that can negatively affect adrenal function over time. Dr. Wilson more specifically describes these stressors that can cause the development of adrenal fatigue, which includes traumatic events, illnesses and simply prolonged, chronic stress from the accumulation of everyday stressors. The book includes line art charts/graphs that depict these stressors and their effects upon the adrenal glands, in lowering the reserves of the stress hormone called "cortisol". This is the hormone that drops to sub-clinically low and sometimes even clinically low levels when adrenal fatigue occurs (also called "adrenal exhaustion" and "hypoadrenia").

I will also mention at this point of this review regarding stressors, that my own case of adrenal fatigue, first surfaced in year 2003, following an approximate two-year period of my being involved in property management. I was managing a 100-unit rental facility, collecting rent from tenants and performing grounds maintenance, in addition to repairs needed on the property, if they didn't require licensed credentials. I refused to hire additional employees, even with a budget that allowed for it and with an obvious need for doing so. I eventually became severely stressed as a result and my adrenal fatigue first surfaced, in addition to my autoimmune thyroid disease, called "Hashimoto's thyroiditis". The hypothyroidism requires daily treatment with a prescribed dose of replacement thyroid hormone however, the associated adrenal fatigue is something that I must continue to treat as-needed and keep close watch on, now over 10 years later, because of its tendency to resurface if I do not take the necessary precautions covered in Dr. Wilson's book.

Chronic Diseases and Syndromes are Associated with Fatigued Adrenals

Dr. Wilson goes on to describe signs and symptoms of adrenal fatigue and points out the fact that "chronic diseases" are commonly associated with the syndrome. These include types of infectious and autoimmune diseases plus other syndromes such as Chronic Fatigue Syndrome and fibromyalgia. I like to point out in my own articles, that thyroid disorders are among the chronic diseases that can trigger adrenal fatigue in some patients that have them. Medical research studies cite "stress" as a participating factor in causing thyroid diseases to manifest and this is especially true of patients who develop Graves' disease – the autoimmune form of hyperthyroidism.

Best Treatments for Adrenal Health are Recommended

Most importantly, Dr. Wilson recommends treatments that can help to resolve adrenal fatigue over time, including safe and effective supplements and lifestyle changes. My local pharmacy carries Dr. Wilson's book on a display at their prescription counter and they also carry the line of supplements he recommends in this book. I will refrain from listing the treatments recommended by Dr. Wilson, so as not to give away the most important part of the book. These treatments are best understood within the context they are presented within the book and they will provide better outcomes for adrenal fatigue patients, if followed in the manner that is recommended for each of them. I highly recommend this book to readers who suffer adrenal fatigue and who are seeking answers for how to effectively treat it.

SECTION EIGHT

Metabolic Problems Caused by Thyroid Disorders

TABLE OF CONTENTS:

1. Hypoglycemia Symptoms and Treatments

Hypoglycemia is a word describing low blood glucose levels. Sugars consumed, become glucose in the body, that is taken into all cells, with the help of insulin, to provide them needed energy.

Hypoglycemia is a condition of low blood glucose. In order for our bodies to function properly, we have to have the proper balance of glucose (blood sugar), which provides us energy to perform our daily activities. Glucose can also rise to abnormally high levels within the body which is referred to as "hyperglycemia", however, within the subheadings that follow, the subject of hypoglycemia will be discussed.

SYMPTOMS OF HYPOGLYCEMIA

Hypoglycemia takes place when the glucose level falls too low to provide that needed energy and as a result, symptoms will occur. The symptoms of hypoglycemia may include the following.

- Weakness
- hunger
- thirst
- nervousness/anxiety
- trembling
- mental fogginess
- headache
- blurred vision
- changes in mood

These flares of symptoms may continue or worsen until glucose levels in the blood are replenished by eating a snack or a meal. Most foods contain a degree of glucose or contain other substances that the body converts into glucose with the help of the liver, so waiting too long to eat between meals can cause varied degrees of hypoglycemia.

Some observers of someone having a mild to moderate hypoglycemic episode, may wonder why "nervousness and anxiety" occurs as part of the symptoms. The reason for this, is due to the body attempting to substitute the low glucose with another hormone that will provide immediate energy (adrenaline), until the proper hormone is provided. Yes, glucose is a hormone, just as adrenaline is and just like thyroid hormones are. It is among the metabolism-providing hormones that are essential to proper bodily functions.

NON-DIABETICS EXPERIENCE HYPOGLYCEMIA

Before advances in medical research over the past few decades, it was believed that hypoglycemia was only experienced by people who were diabetics. Doctors now know that other factors can contribute to hypoglycemia in people who are in early stages of developing diabetes (pre-diabetic) and even in people who are not in the process of developing diabetes. Terms used for people who are showing signs of developing diabetes, include "impaired glucose intolerance" and "insulin resistance".

Other potential causes of hypoglycemia include pregnancy, excessive exercise, fasting, certain medications and a reaction to alcohol intolerance. Some people also experience a form of low blood glucose called "reactive hypoglycemia," which occurs after they consume foods high in carbohydrates or sugar content. For reasons not fully understood, excessive sugar consumption in these individuals causes an overreaction by their pancreas -- the endocrine gland that secretes insulin to convert glucose into energy. When this happens too quickly, there is a spike in energy, followed by an episode of reactive hypoglycemia.

AVOIDING HYPOGLYCEMIA AND TREATING IT WHEN IT OCCURS

Avoiding high glucose foods and refined sugars (a low glycemic diet) can help keep blood levels of glucose from dropping suddenly. Eating foods that also contain protein can help the body to better metabolize the glucose contained in foods, at a slower, more even pace. Eating smaller, more frequent meals can also help keep blood glucose at more steady levels, plus eating occasional healthy snacks between meals to help with energy levels in the body that may drop between meals. Avoiding excessive caffeine and alcohol can also help keep glucose levels better balanced because these chemicals are stimulants that can spike glucose levels in the body, causing a sudden drop in the levels afterward. Exercise also helps keep blood glucose at proper levels because it aids in converting glucose into energy, so that it is used by the body at a steady pace.

HYPOGYLCEMIA SHOULD BE CHECKED BY A DOCTOR

While many people who experience occasional episodes of hypoglycemia are not in danger of developing diabetes, it can still be a potential sign of its later development and should be reported to a doctor when experienced. Proper testing can then be ordered so that diabetes can be ruled-out or diagnosed as early as possible and so that treatment can be recommended by a specialized doctor, such as an endocrinologist. People who experience severe episodes of hypoglycemia may pass out and, in these cases, should also be given immediate medical care by a licensed professional. Emergency medical bracelets are sometimes assigned to patients with diabetes or who are at risk for experiencing severe hypoglycemic episodes.

In most cases hypoglycemia is not life-threatening and by incorporating the proper preventative measures to lessen the frequency and severity of episodes, people who have a tendency toward being hypoglycemic, can live normal, quality lives. According to the Mayo Clinic, these same preventative measures can help to avoid diabetes in people who are at risk for developing it.

2. Hypothyroidism and Fatty Liver Disease

Fat cells can build within the livers of people with hypothyroidism, especially in those who are untreated or under-treated with thyroid hormone replacement therapy.

People with one metabolic disorder, including thyroid disease are at higher risk for developing other metabolic disorders and diseases. For example, a patient with hypothyroidism is at increased risk for developing Metabolic Syndrome (a pre-diabetes condition), Adult Onset Diabetes and Adrenal Syndromes/Diseases. This is especially true if the thyroid disease a patient has is the autoimmune type. A low functioning thyroid gland also places an affected person at risk for fat build up in the liver or what is also referred to as "Non-Alcoholic Fatty Liver Disease" (NAFLD). The condition can occur in thyroid patients, as well as in a large percent of the general population (especially in the obese). This disease is metabolic-related because the body is storing an excessive amount of fat in the liver, rather than converting more of it into energy needed by the body. A major reason this occurs, is due to over-consumption of fats and sugars, combined with obesity and the inability of the liver to keep up with the demand for conversion of these into energy.

When the liver becomes overwhelmed in this performance of duty, it instead begins to store more fat. Over time, this can cause inflammation in the liver and increased liver cell damage (hepatic response or "steatosis hepatitis"). Over time can also cause lesions in the liver or "liver sclerosis". While most cases of fatty liver do not lead to actual hepatitis or sclerosis, it is a risk people with the condition should be aware of. They can then address the problem by undertaking diet and lifestyle changes, in order to keep the condition under control and to possibly reverse it or even resolve it over time. Most cases of fatty liver disease are caused by alcohol consumption and since the type being addressed in this article is not this type, the "non-alcoholic" prefix is used. It is true however that despite it being non-alcohol related, people with the non-alcoholic type are highly advised to avoid alcohol consumption, which can worsen the disease.

What are some other ways to help control and possibly resolve NAFLD that some statistics state may affect up to one-third of the population? As is recommended for most metabolic disorders and diseases, patients need to incorporate a healthy regimen of exercise and weight loss/control into their schedules. Even if this means simply walking for 20 minutes at least three times per week. Patients should also avoid fatty foods and refined sugars which both can be stored as fat in the liver. Eating more fruits and vegetables and foods containing high fiber content, can also help with this disease. It is also important to lose weight when you are carrying extra pounds, especially that which accumulates in the mid-section of the body (belly fat).

Most people have no physical symptoms of this disease, although the most common symptoms reported are fatigue and dull pain on the right side of the abdomen, just under the rib cage. NAFLD is usually found incidentally when a patient is blood-tested via a metabolic panel that includes liver function tests. Their liver enzymes will be mildly to moderately elevated (ALT, SGPT and/or AST levels). Once these abnormal liver counts are found, an ultrasound imaging of the liver is performed to confirm fatty infiltration of the liver. If you are a thyroid disease patient, or one that has Metabolic Syndrome or Diabetes, a "Metabolic Panel" including liver function tests should be performed via blood testing, once a year to detect possible development of fatty liver disease. If the disorder is detected, a doctor may prescribe a treatment plan like the one I previously described but statin and anti-diabetic medications may also be prescribed in some cases.

3. Hypothyroidism and Metabolic Syndrome

Diseases, disorders and syndromes affecting bodily metabolism, often manifest together in people who have them. This is also true of hypothyroid patients, who are at risk for Metabolic Syndrome.

There are many co-morbid endocrine disorders that can affect thyroid patients. One of those is a syndrome affecting the body's metabolism, causing it to become slowed-down, called "Metabolic Syndrome". According to reputable medical sources, this syndrome affects millions of people and places them at higher risk for developing diabetes, heart disease and other potentially serious health problems. The syndrome has gained recognition because of its ability to significantly increase the risk for diabetes especially, and in past years it was known by other names including "Syndrome X".

Medical research conclusions for studies of thyroid patients, link the Metabolic Syndrome to thyroid dysfunction, including one by The Journal of Clinical Endocrinology & Metabolism, which is titled "Thyroid Function is Associated with Components of the Metabolic Syndrome in Euthyroid Subjects". In this article, they associate the syndrome to sub-clinical thyroid disease and in hypothyroid patients whose hormones have been corrected back to Euthyroid states (normalized with hormonal replacement therapies). The study states that patients who meet the scenario of having both corrected-hypothyroidism and Metabolic Syndrome, have increased cardiac risks as well.

What is significant about this study, is the fact that most hypothyroid patients who are later treated, will first experienced long-standing, sub-clinical hypothyroidism, before progressing to overt (full blown) hypothyroidism. This means most of us who are diagnosed with hypothyroidism, were at risk for Metabolic Syndrome, even before we were treated for our hypothyroid hormonal imbalances. This can also mean that we carried that risk over, into our early treatment period and some of us may continue to retain the risk for Metabolic Syndrome, despite optimal hypothyroid treatment. This depends on whether we maintain a healthy body weight, proper diet and engaged in adequate exercise, to help our thyroid treatments continue correcting our slowed metabolisms.

Signs and symptoms of Metabolic syndrome may include the following.

- Obesity – from moderate to morbid

- high cholesterol and/or triglycerides

- cravings for foods high in refined sugars and carbohydrates

- fatigue and depressed mood (or anxiety)

- lack of exercise and low motivation for activities

- hypertension or highly fluctuating blood pressure

- insulin resistance and impaired glucose tolerance

Some doctors will diagnose the syndrome, even if a patient doesn't display all these signs and symptoms. In some cases, obesity and slightly elevated glucose levels (insulin resistance), merit the diagnosis by some physicians. Others may diagnose it if a patient has only hypertension and hypercholesterolemia (high cholesterol levels).

With hypothyroid diseases placing those who are treated for them, at higher risk for developing the Metabolic Syndrome, they would do themselves a great service, to keep their body weight at healthy levels and to observe diet plans that lower their carbohydrates. They should also strictly-limit refined sugars and incorporate an exercise plan of aerobic activity into their regimen, for at least one-hour average, per week. Walking is a well-tolerated form of aerobic exercise, that is usually gentle to the joints, that does not require special gear -- other than proper shoes and that can be done just about anywhere. If significant obesity or joint problems are present however, a stationary exercise bike, might be an alternative to consider.

Medical sources state that exercise should be a regimen of at least 1 hour per week. That's about 20 minutes, three days per week, however, some people who walk for example, will make sure they get one hour and forty five minutes of the exercise weekly, which averages fifteen minutes each day of the week (7 X 15 = 1 hour and 45 minutes). The important thing regarding exercise, is that it is undertaken slowly and increased gradually over time, so that it is well-tolerated. People who are elderly, who are extremely obese or who have heart conditions of any type, should first check with their doctors, before starting any exercise routine, including walking.

Metabolic Syndrome need not be a chronic condition or one that leads to a more serious disease affecting the metabolism. Acting early by changing the necessary lifestyles (intervention), can prevent the need for medical treatments that in some cases are required lifelong.

4. Preventing Diabetes in Thyroid Patients

Type 2 Diabetes is also called Adult Onset Diabetes and affects an estimated 15 million Americans. It is more common in adults ages 45 and over and more common in people with other endocrine disorders, including thyroid diseases. There are two basic steps that can be taken to reduce your risk of experiencing the onset of this disease that causes a dysfunction in the way your body metabolizes your blood sugar (glucose), as I discuss below.

STEP ONE: Avoid weight gain and excessively high blood glucose, by being faithful to a diet low in refined sugars (low glycemic diet). Refined sugars are those that do not come naturally but are processed sugars used to manufacture junk foods, such as cakes, cookies, candies, pies and soft drinks. Consuming too much refined sugar, not only causes excess weight gain but over time, can also cause the body to lose its ability to regulate that sugar via the hormone called insulin. This hormone that is released by the pancreas, helps metabolize (convert) the sugar we consume, into energy for the body and helps carry that energy to every cell within the body.

Without adequate glucose in the blood, our organs do not function properly and one major organ that is highly dependent upon glucose is the brain. There is however a limit to how much glucose the body can metabolize and when there is a continual excess of it, it is converted into fat and carbohydrates, and stored in the body. Over time, this causes weight gain and an inability of the body to continue converting the excess amounts of glucose being consumed and at this point, a person may develop a condition called "insulin resistance", a pre-diabetic condition that over time has the potential to become full blown diabetes.

STEP TWO: Incorporate adequate exercise into your weekly schedule, which helps to keep your weight down and helps the body to metabolize glucose properly. Exercise is essential in helping to burn calories and fat in the body, so that less of it is stored. Exercise also helps the body to build muscle tissue from the things we eat, rather than inactivity which contributes to the body storing more fat.

Exercise also helps the body by circulating the hormones that are active in the blood stream and that contribute to our health, energy and metabolism, including insulin which regulates our blood glucose levels. Even mild exercise such as walking for 20 minutes, three or more times a week, can help the body with metabolism and prevention of weight gain and can also contribute to weight loss when a diet plan as discussed in STEP ONE is also in place.

People at risk for diabetes and those who have become diabetic, are told to be faithful to these two steps and they are told these things so often, that they become tired of hearing them. My belief, however, is that when they understand better, the reasons why these two endeavors for health are so important, they tend to take them more seriously. As the saying goes, "Knowledge is Power" and there is power in understanding why these two major life-habits are so very important to metabolic health!

5. Tweaking Diabetic Prevention in Thyroid Patients

Since thyroid disease patients are at higher risk for diabetes, they must make it a priority to tweak their diabetes prevention plan, the best possible. Following below, I will mention a couple of things that are sometimes neglected by people who are at risk for becoming diabetics but that should be adhered-to strictly, to achieve best preventative measures success.

Getting regular checkups by your doctor and monitoring your glucose levels regularly, especially if diabetes runs in your family, is important. It is a good idea for everyone to get yearly checkups by their doctor but if one or both of your parents, or one of your siblings has diabetes, this becomes even more important. Diabetes, like other endocrine diseases (glandular), can run in families and if a close relative has diabetes, you are at a significantly increased risk for developing the disease yourself. Early prevention is the key to avoiding this potentially serious disease, which upon experiencing the onset of, also places a person at higher risk for heart disease. Diabetic people can also eventually experience kidney failure and glaucoma if they do not follow treatment plans properly. Glaucoma is an eye disorder that can eventually lead to diminished eyesight and even blindness.

There are also home glucose monitors available, that allow a person to check their own blood glucose levels regularly, in the convenience of their home. A person at risk for diabetes can check their glucose level at different times of the day and keep a record of their readings, so that they can detect any pattern or change in their glucose regulation and report these changes to their doctor.

Avoiding alcohol or only consuming it in cautious moderation, should be a priority. People at risk for diabetes or who have diabetes are cautioned to avoid alcohol if possible or to at least drink it in low moderation. Alcohol reacts very quickly in the body and your body depends on your liver to clear the alcohol from your system because it is recognized by the body as a toxin. When you drink alcohol, the liver will not function as well at that time, in converting glucose into carbohydrates and fat because it is busy clearing the body of alcohol. This results in a spike or increase in glucose levels in the blood. People who are on insulin shots to treat their diabetes or on an oral medication can seriously hinder the effectiveness of their medication, through alcohol consumption and this is especially true when they consume alcohol on an empty stomach or in excessive amounts.

The liver and the hormone "insulin", both work in the body to regulate glucose, the liver being the organ that converts it into fat and carbohydrates or "stored energy" and insulin being the hormone that converts it into "immediate energy" for the cells of the body (metabolism). By also maintaining a low glycemic diet (one low in carbohydrates and refined sugars) and by incorporating regular aerobic exercise into your health regimen -- even mild exercise (like walking at least 1 hour per week), you can prevent Adult Onset Diabetes -- also called "Type II Diabetes", from developing.

(END)

Approx. 70,360 words in length

Author Bio: Now age 57, as of year-2020, I have background in successful invention marketing and patenting in the 1990s. I received royalties for a time from an invention, that was a spin-off from our main invention (these others were sold out-right). I relate my full story on the subject regarding my main invention ("Rod Floaters"- Co-Inventor: Johnny W. Hall) and advise other inventors on invention licensing and marketing This is in my book titled: "Preparing Inventions for Marketing Success". Within the book I relate the fact that I self-marketed some of my inventions for a time, getting them into Wal-Marts (regionally) and into Bass Pro Shops, who has carried the product for 28 years (since 1992 - the current year 2020), under our product name and eventually in their own packaging and product-name. They now have their own version, many years following our own patent expiration. Also, from year 2006 to present, The Rod Floater has been marketed by TTI-BLAKEMORE, Inc., who paid us sales-royalties, far beyond our patent expiration. Earlier, I was featured in the May/June 2001 issue of Inventors Digest magazine for coming up with the new flotation product idea and patenting it in 1992. I have many free articles that are on the invention marketing subject and other subjects but my Amazon books and audios for purchase, are by far my best resources. NOTE: TTI-Blakemore is now sole owner of The Rod Floater, along with any connected product we previously owned, regarding fishing rod flotation, including its trademark, any improvements, etc... .

I am a graduate of Liberty University (1996) for completion of theological studies. Bible studies are one of my most-covered books-subjects. I am, however, careful to only address those subjects I believe God has given me correct revelation on. I was a Christian Youth Minister, beginning in the 1980s for approximately 20 years (between youth ministries I served in other church capacities as well). I was also a guest speaker to churches, who invited me to present important Bible teachings to their evangelical congregations, during those same years. I am a redeemed man, who has received salvation by acceptance of Jesus Christ and what he did for me in shedding his blood and dying for me on the cross and in his resurrection from the dead, giving me the promise of eternal life, purely by grace (not due to anything I have done, other than to accept it freely).

Most of my other published written works have been about health disorders/diseases. I literally researched 1,000s of hours in order to compile the best possible information for them in my own words, that could fit into 6,000 to 12,000 word-length books, that are exclusive to Amazon; as are all others I have written. I do, however, have some that are much longer. Most people who are ill with these diseases are not looking for lengthy dissertations, in order to obtain the most important information that most laypersons are seeking (non-medical professionals, who are patients). Very few doctors have time to thoroughly educate their patients. The reputable information that is available online, usually requires searching multiple sites to find all the abridged, full-spectrum, layperson information needed by uninformed patients. I have studied these resources and medical manuals, to compile my books into relate-able resources for fellow patients.

When you are seriously ill, lengthy online search is not always the preferred option. Hopefully that statement will help those readers out there, complaining of layperson authors, covering medical information in books and articles. Especially with medical errors being the 3rd leading cause of death in the USA. I certainly hope it does because many of us who do so, have spent many years gleaning the best possible information to share with fellow patients. Mary Shomon for example, is the Nation's #1 Thyroid Disease Advocate and she has no medical credentials. She has however, written several New York Times Best Sellers on thyroid disease.

One somewhat controversial book I published is titled: "Effects of UNFAIRLY UNFAVORABLE Book Reviews on Independent Authors" (there is no attack language whatsoever in the book). The book was an experiment of sorts and I stated this fact on the Amazon KDP forum in advance of publishing it. It points out problems with authors as well as with reviewers. I made it very clear in the book, that I was not talking about unfavorable reviews but "unfairly unfavorable reviews", meaning those containing overboard/excessive "attack language". As stated above, the book makes negative points about authors as well as it does about reviewers. I have never directed comments directly at reviewers (specific people). I have responded to comments posed to me as questions but very few times.

Additionally, I added some comedy to the rhetoric via my books titled: "Bashing Authors with Negative Reviews and Feeling Fully Justified" (written via my pen name: Fredrick Doyle Wimberly) and "Writing Books That Won't Get Blue Meanie Reviews" (via my pen name "Percyvelle Pennington III"). Many readers understood the purpose for these other books, which was to add a bit of comedy to the reviewer/author wars, with hopes that it would lighten the hostility a little. Readers of these comedy-shorts, added a number of 5-star reviews to them, containing great comments and of the 9 reviews the "Blue Meanies Reviews" one has received for example, I only provided free review copies to 2 of the reviewers. I do not know the other reviewers who were highly favorable toward to book, either online or in person. I also compiled all three titles together, being titled: "Wars Between Book Reviewers and Authors" and one 5-star review has already been expressed with noted understanding of the purpose of it. I also do not know the writer of this nice-length favorable review, online or in person.

In late 2002 - early 2003, I experienced a severe illness. I was first diagnosed with autoimmune thyroid disease and co-morbid Chronic Fatigue Syndrome/Fibromyalgia. My illness worsened despite treatment for 'the thyroid disease aspect of it' and it was manifesting like a neurological disease. My employment at the time, required considerable commuting-driving and I eventually reached a point that my legs and feet were not working well enough to drive more than short distances. All of this is detailed in my health subject books. I worked for 8 years after the illness onset, all the while getting repeat MRIs, ultrasounds, heart tests, spinal taps, etc... A neurologist eventually recommended "vitamin E" blood testing and I had less than a half-point in my body ("0.4"). It was because of my neuro-pain and muscle weakness, etc.... that he decided on that test. Hole punch biopsies and nerve conduction studies already showed large and small fiber peripheral neuropathies (damaged nerves).

I wrote and published books for each of the medical conditions I have experienced, including asthma, non-smoker COPD, NAFLD, heart disease plus for other related health conditions. In year- 2012, I began receiving permanent medical disability benefits. I also wrote a book on this subject and if you're familiar with SSDI, they pay less than one's former occupation. However, thank the Good Lord for the medical benefits because the medical care probably saved my life or at least has extended it until I'm of old age. This is not a guarantee but I'm believing God for it. I'm open to supernatural healing as well (divine intervention), in God's sovereign timing and will. I have witnessed God's supernatural intervention during my life, and I write about this in my book titled: "God Performs Supernatural Works Today".

My book proceeds became far more important to me due to my illnesses. I also began writing at every chance to inform others on these and other subjects I see great importance in. With exception of my comedy titles, which are purely for enjoyment. I could also see how important it was for fellow writers I became acquainted with on fellow patient forums, to protect their written works, some of which have died since I came to know them only a few years ago (one in-particular committed suicide, due to their illness). Seeing our books as "our babies", as some bloggers, have accused me and other writers of? No, not exactly but we do see them as possible highly needed support for others. I believe my battles are fought by the Lord as I move forward (2 Chronicles 20:15). I also believe we will all reap from the things we are sowing in this life, to help or to harm others- (Galatians 6:7).

It is my sincere hope that those who are interested in the subjects I offer in my books, will truly benefit from the information contained within them.

Best Regards and God Bless,

James M. Lowrance